About the Author

Sylvia Bryden-Stock is an holistic coach and healer blessed to love her wonderful husband against all odds. She had a successful nursing and business career, working in the community as a district nurse. Managing a care home has given her an insight into dementia and Alzheimers disease and a connection to the different services available at that time.

Broadening her spiritual outlook on life and her personal development formulated a move from her narrow restricted beliefs, to a belief in the oneness of all things, and the power of the divinity or consciousness that lies within all of us.

It is her background and, most of all, her spiritual awareness that has helped with the personal journey she is still on with her beloved husband.

Sylvia's life has taken many twists and turns that have become her greatest teachers and the catalyst for spiritual and personal growth. Through her coaching and healing programme, it is her passion to help others find their inner 'consciousness self' and allow that to guide daily earthly life experiences.

It is this approach to life that has so helped on the journey you are about to embark upon.

The Rocky Road of Naughty Neurons

Our Journey with Young Onset Alzheimer's Disease

Sylvia Bryden-Stock
RGN ONC SCM NDN Health Ed Cert
Reiki Master Dip Crystal Healing
Transformational Coach & Speaker

Book Guild Publishing

First published in Great Britain in 2016 by
The Book Guild Ltd
9 Priory Business Park
Wistow Road, Kibworth
Leicestershire, LE8 0RX
Freephone: 0800 999 2982
www.bookguild.co.uk
Email: info@bookguild.co.uk
Twitter: @bookguild

Copyright © 2016 Sylvia Bryden-Stock

The right of Sylvia Bryden-Stock to be identified as the author of this
work has been asserted by her in accordance with the
Copyright, Design and Patents Act 1988.

All rights reserved. No part of this publication may be
reproduced, transmitted, or stored in a retrieval system, in any form or by any means,
without permission in writing from the publisher, nor be otherwise circulated in
any form of binding or cover other than that in which it is published and without
a similar condition being imposed on the subsequent purchaser.

Typeset in Hoefler

Printed and bound in Great Britain by
CPI Group (UK) Ltd, Croydon, CR0 4YY

ISBN 978 1 91087 828 6

British Library Cataloguing in Publication Data.

A catalogue record for this book is available from the British Library.

Contents

	Acknowledgements	vii
	Introduction	ix
1	'Fate' or 'Coincidence'?	1
2	'Deceit' or 'Necessary Clarification'?	7
3	The Nightmare Becomes a Reality	12
4	The Journey Begins – Emotions and Frustrations	16
5	Coping with Emotions, Frustrations; Letting go	20
6	Brian's Perspective	29
7	Finding the Blessings?	38
8	Suddenly the Rocks on the Road Appear	44
9	Yes You Can!	53
10	Get me to the Church on Time!	61
11	A Scary Honeymoon	71
12	Life is Somewhat Settled	76
13	Oh my! What is Happening Now? The Blue Badge Scenario	86
14	We Did Have Clear Cut Goals!	92
15	A Holiday – Well Sort of!	99
16	A Change in Challenges – Letting Go?	112
17	24/7 Care – A Journey of Its Own	120
18	Integration – A Holistic Approach	128
19	Some Suggestions from Sylvia	133
	In Summary	137
	References	138

Acknowledgements

I wish to dedicate this book to my darling husband, who so bravely accepted the diagnosis and the implications that had for the pending journey. I love you for your approach to this drastic change in our life together.

Thank you to the consultant Dr. Jonathan Robbin, who so sensitively announced the diagnosis, and for his support for our desire to holistically approach the ensuing journey we faced.

Thank you to the local Alzheimer's Society, who were so supportive as I struggled with researching what I knew one day soon would be Brian's diagnosis. Also, blessings to you for 'being there' at times when I needed help to cope in the earlier days.

Thank you to Brian's local GP, who was always so kind and understanding when we visited for appointments, and for his prompt referral after our first very painful visit. He must have had his own feelings of sadness, as he had known Brian for many years through Brian holding regular barn dances at his son's school.

Thank you to the family and friends who have been there for us with unquestioning care and support, kind words, encouragement and healing prayers.

Thanks goes to our lawyer, who so successfully helped us achieve our goal of being married.

Thank you to all the wonderful staff at Princess Christian Care Home in Knaphill, Surrey, who give what I consider five star care to my darling husband.

Thank you to the angels and that 'God' essence of Sylvia, which has helped during some of the darkest moments on this rocky road.

Introduction

Suddenly realising that your partner could potentially have Alzheimer's disease is a major blow, even when we have a deep spiritual faith and are living an holistic lifestyle as a transformational coach and healer.

Believe me, no matter how much you have learned through life's experiences, with the tools and skills that you share with others seeking to transform their lives, this earthly journey can throw up some very interesting experiences.

Life experiences have much to teach us, enabling us to grow within our soul, and giving greater understanding to what others are going through as they journey through their own challenges.

I recall a time of my life when I volunteered to be the first aid nurse for an organisation called Interact, based in Walton-on-Thames in Surrey. Every Tuesday at the end of school, both mainstream and learning disability children came together for two and a half hours to participate in drama and music. Of course, I met the parents of the learning disability children and was in awe at how much love they had for their child. It was evident that there was a good bond between them, and some of the parents actually said they would not change things, having come through the initial shock after the baby was born.

I was truly humbled by this experience, which lasted two and a half years. Leaving the role due to my holistic career talking off was heart-wrenching, as I had grown to really bond with many of the children, and would be greeted every week with big hugs from the Down's Syndrome children. One epileptic teenager in particular would throw her arms around me and nearly break my ribs with the power of the hug!

Why do I relate this time in my life? It shows how, with inner determination and deep love for someone who develops a very challenging condition, you can find ways to cope with the ups and downs of day-to-day life. It is important as the carer to look after oneself, and as you journey with Sylvia and Brian through their journey, you will realise how honesty, coupled with our deep love for each other, has stood the test of time so far on the Alzheimer's path.

You will also see how Sylvia faced her own grief and had to learn to care for herself first in order to best care for the man she loved and married during the earlier stages of his condition. There is still much to learn about Alzheimer's, so I will also share some thoughts on an holistic approach to helping someone when diagnosed.

Brian has a unique manifestation of Alzheimer's disease as he has also been diagnosed with Posterior Cortex Atrophy – more about that in the story, including what it is in lay terms and the added challenges it causes.

There lies deep within all of us a higher self that will guide us through the darkest of experiences. It is by drawing on that part of me on our journey that I have come through thus far, developing strategies of peace and a knowing that I cannot walk my husband's path for him. Nor should I feel guilty about "Should I have done any more to hold this journey back?"

May our story help you on your journey – as Eckhart Tolle, author and speaker, so aptly put it:

"Realise deeply that the present moment is all you have. Make the NOW the primary focus of your life."

CHAPTER ONE

'Fate' or 'Coincidence'?

It was a typical Sunday evening. Sylvia lived on her own in Woking in a downstairs, one-bedroom flat, having left her partner of ten years. There had been an engagement and potentially pending marriage until it was finally realised that his past marriage partner was still 'in control'. The parting of the ways was traumatic, yet with grit and determination, Sylvia moved on to focus her attention on work and her spiritual calling.

Evenings out to typical singles clubs left her disillusioned with the opposite sex, and thoughts of ever meeting someone 'on the same wavelength' seemed almost impossible.

So here we are at 6.15 p.m. contemplating whether to attend the local spiritualist church service, only minutes away, or stay at home. Something within spurred on the decision to go to the service. Sylvia quickly donned smart clothing and preened herself – makeup and hair to perfection – got in her car and speedily drove the short distance. Just in time, it was a back row seat that was left. The service involved a visiting speaker and medium, who would give inspiring messages from loved ones and the angelic world beyond. This particular night it was a local gentleman, and as he walked down to the front of the room and sat down, the thought was 'Cor! He's nice! Probably married with the statutory 2.8 kids!' I recall him coming to me during his mediumship demonstration and giving me an accurate and encouraging message, which also impressed.

At the end of the service tea and biscuits were served. As Sylvia indulged a voice seemed to say to her 'Go and talk to the medium' (Sylvia also has a gift of channelling and knew it was an inspired thought coming in). Getting up from her seat at the back of the venue, Sylvia went down with her cup of tea and sat by the medium and thanked him for the message. Conversation ensued and Sylvia talked about her own spiritual gifts she was blessed to work with.

What then followed was what has been described many times since as the best chat up line ever received in Sylvia's life.

"You know, us mediums never seem to get messages for ourselves."

"Really!" was the immediate reponse.

"Here's my card. I'll give you a reading sometime if you like."

Time was passing, so Sylvia got up, said goodbye and headed home to meet up later with a friend to discuss progress with their network marketing business. No real thought was given to the handsome gentleman she had met earlier.

Smart clothes were exchanged for comfortable casual for the rest of the evening. It was barely ten minutes since arriving home when the telephone rang.

"Hello?" The usual guarded response to calls and ready to field unwanted marketing calls was given, but the voice at the end of the telephone was none other than the man she had met earlier at the church!

"Hello, it's Brian here! I was really enjoying our conversation, can we meet and continue it?"

"Sorry, I have a friend coming round now, but would love to meet during the week and talk over a coffee or drink." He is obviously single, was my immediate, happy thought!

"When are you free?" I asked. "I could meet on Wednesday."

"Sorry, I go to folk club on Wednesday."

"How about Friday or Saturday?" was the eager request.

"No, I am a barn dance caller with my own band and am busy both nights."

After a good few minutes checking our diaries a date was arranged for two weeks later. Nothing like keeping a man waiting, eh!

I remember our very first official date very well. He picked me up in his company car, and was dressed smart/casual, as thankfully was I. Off we went to a local pub just outside Woking town centre, where it was karaoke night. I soon learned that Brian was an avid folk fan, and had been given voice training in his youth.

"Do you sing?" he asked.

"Well, I enjoy singing and was in a school choir, and I also sang a lot at church whilst playing the guitar," I responded, trying to impress as best I could.

We were given a list of all the songs available and Brian confidently got up and sang his first song. What it was I cannot now recall, except I remember thinking, 'Wow! He's even got a sexy singing voice!'

He returned to sit beside me and encouraged me to get up and sing. 'Oh my! Hope I can impress,' I thought.

Nervously, I got up and sang Edelweiss from the *Sound of Music*, which got a rapturous round of applause *and* impressed my date! He sang a second song and, on returning to his seat, asked if I was going to sing again. Scanning the list I couldn't find a song that would be easily performed. Suddenly this voice beside me snapped, "Come on Sylvia. Hurry up and choose!"

Well, in that moment I had a split-second feeling that perhaps I wouldn't go out again with a man who was so belittling to me. I decided I would sing *Hey There, Georgie Girl* by the New Seekers, and got up to sing. Halfway through the first verse I had a coughing fit and had to give up on the song. Immense relief came over me as I sat down. Fortunately there were no more snappy remarks during the rest of the evening, and I was propelled home to my door. 'No – he is not coming in on first date,' was my thought, and so he left, though we did agree to meet again. He was what one might say the 'perfect gentleman' with dating, and not rushing to have any intimate contact, which impressed me.

As time went on we grew to be close friends and I knew I wanted to develop a strong relationship with him. Time together was fitted around my agency nursing, network marketing activities and spiritual work, plus his daily business routine, barn dances – he had his own band – and also his spiritual work.

This continued as a loving relationship and we became strongly committed as partners. We never really discussed marriage as it transpired that Brian had been through a very challenging marriage and was not keen to re-marry. I too had nearly married twice and felt that a strong partnership was better than facing commitment and creating the potential for a sad ending to a wonderful, deeply loving relationship. We have both agreed many times that it is like we are expressing 'divine love' through and to each other.

Life continued with us growing stronger together with that deep love flowing between us. I remember being a part of the barn dance band as his 'demonstrator'. Having been in a school country-dance team and won a trophy, I was definitely up for going along when first invited, and built a strong friendship with the band. Typically, a blessing in our relationship was our ability to love each other for who we are, and a desire to be on this earthly journey and not to control it. For me, true love and strong relationships survive by allowing the love to express itself around life commitments and personal choices without judgement.

The years went on and family and friends could see the depth of our love for each other. Never, ever did we think that this love would be tested to such limits as it has been...

CHAPTER TWO

'Deceit' or 'Necessary Clarification'?

Life was great and we were happy sharing our life together until around the early millennia years, when little things like small general money problems and phone calls from the barn dance band members began. They were concerned about Brian, as he was not arriving to gigs as punctually as usual, as well as seeming to have got lost on the way at times. A very disciplined man who expected things to run like clockwork, he was becoming confused with the handling of the money at the end of the evening, as well as repeating dance calls or giving the wrong instructions. These things were so out of character with a man who had successfully managed barn dance gigs for almost thirty years.

Typical phone calls to me on evenings when I was not with him were, "Has Brian left yet? We are worried. He should have been here by now." The most concerning evening I experienced was a Friday, when a gig had been arranged in a church hall, which I believe was not one of his usual venues. My phone rang and it was one of the band members. "Has Brian left? It's time we started."

I said that he would certainly be on his way and asked that they try to keep in touch. By now the band were bringing extra gear to gigs as back up if he was late. I was assured I would be kept in the picture.

Time passed and I received another call that he was now an hour late, and they were coping with the running of things. This now triggered concern in me and I went round to a friend's for tea and calming down. Had he had an accident? Where on earth could he be?

By 10 p.m. he had still not arrived at the gig, and I was ready to phone hospitals in the area and even the police. Suddenly my friend, who is very intuitive, said, "Do you know, I think he is at home. I don't know why, but let's try his phone number."

"Ok," I nervously responded, and with a sick feeling in my solar plexus dialled Brian's number.

"Hello," said a normal voice.

"What are you doing at home? The band are worried about you!" I retorted.

Totally out of character, the reply was, "Well there were about five churches in the area and I couldn't f*****g well find the right one so in the end I came home!"

"Why didn't you call the band?" was my almost angry reply.

"Well, I knew that they would be getting on with the evening," he stated, as if there was nothing to be concerned about, and he seemed surprised that I was ready to put out calls to hospitals and the police.

I immediately called the band and let them know what had happened, after which I went round to his home and we spent the night together. I later learned that he would call the event organiser four or five times to get directions, which was not really very professional. At work – he was a sales rep – he began to leave his diary at his customers' or sometimes take the incorrect information file – an unheard of thing with his almost over-the-top precision and discipline. When driving with Brian, I began to notice little things like distance and speed judgement, and was a little uneasy at times as a passenger. Our guardian angel must have been looking after us as we had no incidents or accidents when out and about. I did sometimes offer to drive my car instead. I quietly suggested that Brian visit his GP, as I was a bit concerned, as was some of his family. He agreed and came back ecstatic as the GP said that his memory was no worse than hers.

Not convinced that this was the case I decided to do some research without his knowledge. You see, my background was nursing and subsequently a care home manager working with residents, some of whom were dementia patients, so I knew the signs.

I began researching on the Internet and contacted the local Alzheimer's Association to arrange a chat with someone. It was suggested that I attend the carer's group on a Tuesday evening. As this was a night where we both did 'domestics' and did not meet up, it was the ideal night. As I met the people each week I soon realised that my fears were a reality, and that it was only time before I would have to face Brian with my concerns and get him to a doctor.

It was not at all easy during this time because it felt like I was being deceitful, which is totally against my moral and spiritual principles. Outwardly I was my usual self, but observing the changes and hurting big time inside, as I knew the time was soon going to loom for a confrontation which could, of course, precipitate total denial and a possible end to a deeply loving, trusting relationship. The Alzheimer's Society were very supportive and were repeatedly telling me to get Brian to see a doctor for a diagnosis. The inner pain was growing and I was literally praying for help in approaching the issue.

One summer's day in 2009 I sat on my sofa with Brian and it was as if an inner something came over me with the courage to broach the subject. Almost tearfully I began to tell him of my concerns and, amazingly, he said he had noticed some challenging things since before the previous Christmas. Relief came over me and together we agreed to get him to see a GP.

"How about we start afresh with another GP in the practice?" I suggested. Luckily there was the GP who had known him for many years – not as his GP – but through Brian's barn dance band doing gigs at his son's school!

So one June morning we arrived at his surgery and we began to tell him emotionally what was going on. Thus began the journey to diagnosis.

CHAPTER THREE

The Nightmare Becomes a Reality

The GP initially arranged blood tests and a urine screening and these came back as not showing any abnormalities. The next referral was to see the elderly care physician who also dealt with dementia patients at our local hospital. Luckily we got an appointment within a three-month period. He was a gentle natured and caring gentleman who started a further chain of events as he wished to 'rule out' such diagnosis as transient ischemic attack (mini strokes) and a brain tumour. The first test was an MRI scan, which had a waiting time of around eight weeks, but we were to be on standby in case of a cancellation. I was being as strong as I possibly could for my man, as one could not imagine what he must have been going through mentally, although he never showed it. Not only was he going through this traumatic time, but in 2001 he was made redundant from work and had not been working since, due to the downturn in the building trade – he sold kitchens to builders and had had a successful career spanning over 20 years.

The MRI appointment came through and I had permission to sit in with him, not only for support, but I wished to experience what went on to be able to better empathise with my coaching clients who may have been through this experience. Brian took it all in his stride and actually said it was not at all unpleasant lying in a cramped tubular space with his head clamped still for 40 minutes. Even the music playing to dull the noise of the scanner did not seem to phase him. A few weeks later we were given a further consultant appointment for the results. We both did a quiet sigh of relief when we were told that there was no sign of stroke or brain tumour. However, another test was then prescribed to check the brain's arterial capacity, known as a SPECT scan. This shows how the blood flows through the arteries in the brain and captures brain activity. A radioactive material (tracer) is injected into the vein in the arm and the scanner detects the movement of the tracer through the brain. Pictures of the brain are taken as the patient lies very still.

This test was done in October 2009, and we had to wait until January 2010 for a follow-up appointment.

I was dreading this one, as somehow I knew this would be the moment of truth for Brian and myself. As we entered the consulting room you could almost, as mother would have said, cut the air with a knife. The consultant did his usual greeting and said, "Well, the good news is that we have now totally ruled out cancer and mini strokes or other tumours. However, I do have some bad news for you, Brian. The SPECT scan shows that you have young onset Alzheimer's disease."

Although I had expected this diagnosis I went numb.

Brian was silent for a few seconds, and then said, "Well, I suppose I will have to do my best to live with it," in a very matter of fact voice – probably because it had not really sunk in.

He then underwent the typical Alzheimer's M.M.S.E. test (Mini Mental State Examination) and scored a total 25/30, which meant he was in the early stages. Aricept 10 mgs, one at night, was prescribed. A consultant prescription only, so we were given a three month prescription to carry us over to the next appointment.

The actual SPECT scan image amazed me as it showed a large area of brain damage and yet there were no drastic signs of the disease at this stage.

As we left the hospital clutching hands, I knew I had to reassure him that I would be with him right through the journey. When you love someone as deeply as I always have, this is not a time to abandon them because of the unknown future ahead. We stopped off at Morrisons on the way home for a coffee, and not a lot was said as we were in shock, in spite of my inner knowing. How grateful I was for the 'homework' I had done. This meant I would now get Brian the support to help live this journey – as well as for myself, of course.

We went home and spent a quiet evening together. It was important that we shared the diagnosis with those dear to us in Brian's own time and not mine. That particular evening is all a bit of a blur as we were obviously in shock – me as well in spite of having the research confirmed. I think I did share with him what I had been doing and how dreadful I felt about 'living a lie'. With him being the sensitive soul that he is, he fully understood and still sees the benefit of what I had done. So here we are preparing – or trying to prepare – for the unknown journey ahead, as everyone expresses this disease in their own unique way within the parameters of how it generally manifests its expression. What now? Where do we begin?

CHAPTER 4

The Journey Begins – Emotions and Frustrations

Having accepted as best we could the truth of what could lie ahead, Brian was determined to do his very best not to let it get him down.

Because he was in the early stages, life pretty much went on as before, with us living in our separate dwellings, but Brian spending more time with me. The local Alzheimer's Society were very supportive at this stage, with a key worker visiting Brian regularly for support and helpful advice. I too had a visit as his carer and was able to offload concerns regarding what I was observing with Brian. Endeavouring to keep life as normal as possible meant that I had to 'turn a blind eye' to things observed that were becoming challenging to Brian from day-to-day due to memory issues manifesting. Also, part of you seems to pretend that things are not really happening, and both of us would be in a state of denial as a coping mechanism. Brian's frustrations with being challenged with day-to-day tasks would be expressed with anger and by saying swear words not used previously.

As an holistic coach and healer, and Brian being a healer, I discussed with him the options of also including an holistic approach to the journey by incorporating both Reiki healings and natural supplements to support general health and feed the brain tissue that were still functioning. Fortunately our consultant was open-minded and encouraged my research and use of natural alternatives, alongside the Aricept drug. This is discussed in a later chapter.

Telling family and friends was a painful and emotional time as it was reinforcing our having to accept the diagnosis as a reality, not just a dream we will wake up from one day.

Being quite an emotional soul, born under the sign of the crab, Cancer, I can cry over anything for joy or sorrow! My way of dealing with what I was observing in Brian, and knowing from my care home manager background the typical journey, was to cry when alone to release the pain. I had and have great friends and family who were there for both of us, plus our spiritual friends were very supportive.

I feel it is important to say here that no two people will grieve on this journey in the same way. There are no specific scripts, only pointers and tips on how to deal with the one diagnosed when certain behaviour manifests itself, that sometimes work and sometimes do not.

Sometimes I would grieve with Brian, reassuring him

of my commitment to see the journey through with him no matter what or how. Brian's way of dealing with his manifestation of the disease was mostly through anger, frustration and depression. He began to use language I had never heard him use before so frequently! One evening he was staying at my place and had brought his DVD player to watch something whilst I got on with other things. Oh dear! His challenges kicked in and he was struggling to put things together. Suddenly his temper rose and he swore, the box went flying across the room. I realised that this could well be how he was going to express his emotions along the way. Thankfully it was only the box that went flying!

We did go through a time where he regularly became angry and aggressive, even towards me, blaming me for being stupid if I could not understand his communicating due to speech/language difficulties. Fortunately, he was not violent towards me in the earlier stages, and I do feel my patient nature plus past experience and spiritual calm has helped here. However, my own personal dilemma in the earlier days was that as I was a coach/healer and believe deeply in the power of the higher self and angels to cope with this earthly journey, I should always be able to be at peace no matter what – to live what I was teaching! As time has gone on I have realised that even the greatest spiritual healers that have walked on earth had their times of suffering and challenge. The Master Jesus got angry at the Pharisees and Sadducees, never mind the day he got angry in the temple and overturned the tables of those selling.

Emotions must be expressed and as carers we have to know that no matter what inner strength we have and a determination to support our loved ones (whether it be partner, spouse, parent etc.), we have to look after ourself first! Not easy, I grant you, but I am learning as I write this book to take care of myself. Yes, it can cause challenges, especially when, with the Alzheimer's journey the patient is more often than not in denial of their challenges, and cannot understand how the carer can be so tired.

This journey has to be lived in each moment. We cannot predict or fully know how the future will play out, even though some planning has to take place for the probable future.

CHAPTER 5

Coping with Emotions, Frustrations; Letting go

Let me try to help readers here from my own experience, as I have vowed with Brian that our journey will be an endeavour that can help others cope on their own journey. You see, Sylvia's life journey has been one of twists and turns, dealing with emotional issues and learning to become more self-empowered, as well as providing an awareness of who we all truly are – emotional energetic expressions of the creative source through the physical form.

It is as if this journey of ours is here to teach us something profound about (certainly as carers) finding and allowing the higher self to help deal with the manifestations we encounter. Easier said than done many times, I can tell you. But let me share with you more about how we deal with our day-to-day life with Alzheimer's.

It is fair to say that emotions that one never thought were part of the Alzheimer's sufferers' make up, suddenly begin to manifest themselves. I can recall from when I worked in the care home industry a typical resident who had held a high position within the Church of England. His character through life had been one of sobriety, and never would a profanity ever be uttered from his mouth. Oh my! How different it was since he had developed a form of dementia. Daily language was far from what one would have expected from a man of the cloth. Initially, family were embarrassed, but in time they adjusted to the new character being manifested. Brian had always been a man who never really swore or got aggressively angry. A few months after diagnosis that changed, and I was faced with a man expressing his frustration at things that began to challenge him by becoming very angry and sometimes directing it at me. Yes, it was scary sometimes. What did I do? Initially I felt fear and was upset as I witnessed this man, who I deeply loved, developing. I would cry when on my own and call on my angels and God to help me cope. There was an absolute feeling of guilt that I was not coping when I totally believed in the power of prayer and inner stillness to bring peace and calm and the ability to cope with situations. All kinds of pain and grief began to emerge, and on good days a total denial, as one could live a normal life. The support worker was a great help as she also had a deep spiritual side to her. This made it easier for me to offload. I used to say to her, "I feel as if I need to talk to The Dalai Lama!"

Over time, Sylvia has learnt that, to truly be a great teacher and healer, we have to fully experience here on earth and release emotions to get to the place of inner peace. I was still able to do regular yoga exercises and meditation, and this helped begin the day with a sense of connection to my peaceful and joyful inner self. A great tool I developed when things began to get more challenging.

Wherever you are, take a deep breath in and say, "I choose peace in this situation" as you breathe out. With consistent practice you can get to a state of inner peace. It is important to work on not getting caught up in a patient's energy as much as possible. They seem to pick up on the carer's negative energy and react.

This journey is a bit like going back to school to relearn life skills. During the earlier phase of Brian's journey, we were able to talk about what was happening and honesty helped greatly. We agreed to call his Alzheimer's manifestations 'naughty neurones'; or "It's those Neurones again!" This helped greatly. By using this terminology it took away any direct personal relationship to Brian alone. Often I would be asked, "What is happening to me?" My response with a hug, would be, "It's those Naughty Neurones again," or "It's those damned Neurones."

We also managed to laugh over some of the challenges on most days. This can be a great way of dissipating a challenging moment. Brian would even tell friends that we "laugh nearly every day."

The importance in the earlier stages of letting Brian struggle with trying to do things was painful to watch, and emotionally it was like trying to tie one's hands behind your back and 'zip the lips', when you wanted to help. I soon learned about this when offering a little help with dressing. Without thinking I said, "But darling, you have challenges and need help with things." Ooops! Wrong! The angry retort was, "No I don't. I've been doing this for years! Are you stupid or something? I can do this!"

With inner pain I stood back and only when he really could not manage his trouser belt or buttons did I quietly do it for him without a word being said, and then gave him a kiss and hug.

I had to get used to toothpaste everywhere in the bathroom where he struggled with his posterior cortex atrophy. Eventually, I began to slowly adjust our morning and bedtime routine in a way that enabled extra help to be given without him getting agitated or upset.

Flexibility is so important on this journey. One day is never the same as another. Many issues are also quite bizarre at times. Just as you think that you have got it sussed with what can be remembered, they recall a recent event with the greatest of clarity. It is as if the neurones still working can 'catch' an event and somehow save it somewhere. Maybe I am blessed with a good deal of patience, but even that has been challenged along the way! Repetition was the watchword all day long, but

I did my best to bring humour into it. I would suddenly laugh and he would ask, "What is so funny?"

"Well, I have lost count of how many times you have asked that," I would say with a smile.

"You are dreaming again!" would be the retort.

"I wish I was," I would reply, and then give him a big hug. We ended up laughing together.

Being quite sensitive should, alongside his stubborn Aquarius temperament, mean that I could sometimes express how it pained me to see his challenges, and how I was in awe of his attempt to maintain a happy attitude. He would then give me a big hug and let me have a tearful release for a few minutes. This was of course in the early-to mid-stages before full time care was needed.

One thing for sure on this journey – it is impossible to fully generalise how it will play out. Everyone manifests their symptoms in different ways at the different stages of the disease. We, as carers, can never be complacent about the journey as our loved one flits between moods and emotions as the brain neurone signals fire off in random patterns according to the areas affected.

For Sylvia, what has been the greatest blessing as our journey progresses is the deep unconditional love we have for each other. Yet this blessing can also cause the greatest pain, as you watch that person change and watch the true personality gradually disappear. The saying 'True love hurts' most certainly is experienced! On fairly good days one can feel that life is as it was before, and be pretty much in carer denial as part of you wants some kind of miracle to take this whole thing away. Then suddenly symptoms show up again and the new reality expresses itself once more. Keeping emotions in check is like trying to balance scales all the time. Not knowing how each moment is going to play out can be very tiring. As the carer you live out the role as best you can. It is so important to find ways to get support for yourself. Yes – easier said than done, very often as the partner is in denial a lot of the time and refuses any outside input or help.

Sylvia's nursing and care home manager background could be said to be a great asset throughout this challenging time. To a certain extent that is true, but in the cold light of day, one is *not* living out a nurse's role. You are another spouse hurting as you see what is happening to the one you so deeply love.

So what have been the major issues for Sylvia on this rollercoaster ride of Alzheimer's disease?

1. The nurse always deals with situations and copes, because that is what she is trained to do. One lives daily, instinctively getting on with what is required to keep the patient cared for and happy, no matter how tired one is, because you have been programmed how to care and give without showing frustration or anger. You just keep on keeping on as if you are still living that role and expect to be able to do it all.

2. As an holistic transformational coach who believes in the power of God, consciousness and angels to see us through challenges, Sylvia has frequently beaten herself up over the fact that to live in inner peace at all times has been difficult. 'I should be able to do this totally from my higher self at all times', is the thought frequently going through my head. Then I will know only that, in truth, all great spiritual teachers and masters needed to experience suffering to prove the power of the 'higher self' within. After all, we are here on earth to experience challenges in many forms. It is through these challenges that we can actually grow as a person.

One very important thing on this road we travel is to come to accept that we must release our feelings as carers and not keep them bottled up. Stress undealt with is the root cause of disease. Science now tells us that over 85% of all illnesses have their roots in stress. Yes, I know from experience, it becomes challenging to find ways to vent emotions as you become more engrossed in the carer's role and coping with see-saw moods in the one you love. I am not ashamed to tell you that I have, from time to time, picked up the phone for a five minute vent with the Samaritans. No, I was not desperate and suicidal. Far from it – I just needed to *release my emotions* and then I could be strong and cope again. I recall one day when I was so full of my own pain and frustrations, at a time when my husband and I would reasonably deal with things as a team, I said to him, "I am just going upstairs to make a phone call. I need to deal with my emotions," as tears welled up.

"Ok," he said. Five minutes later he had a smiling wife back. We hugged and carried on with our day, with Sylvia better able to cope with him.

In the early stages of Alzheimer's communication is key to help prevent anger outbursts from the patient, which are of course due to their own frustrations. I have lost count of the times Brian has said to me, "I have been able to do this all my life – why can't I do it now?" This is where using the phrase I wrote earlier, 'naughty neurones', comes in. I would usually respond with, "It's those crazy naughty neurones that get mixed up." This seemed to dissipate what could have become an angry scene.

To all you lovely carers out there reading this book, I want to tell you that one of the biggest challenges we face is guilt about not always being able to cope, guilt when the patient 'throws a major wobbly'. How could I have prevented this? We have to let go of guilt and know that we are doing the very best we can in the circumstances. *There is no logical formula for success on this journey.* Yes, there are guidelines about how behaviour manifests due to the challenges in neurone activity in the patient's brain, and very useful information on how best to deal with anger outbursts and denial. Then there is our view of the world and our own past experiences that influence our responses to what happens in our world, which are influenced by past programming in formative years. Some people are blessed with a greater level of patience by their own character make up. Others are more outspoken and forthright. Both traits are OK, and have their benefits on this journey. Maybe patience will minimise outbursts from the patient, as one is able to be more calm as one's whole world is changing around you. Then one might say, does the patience also mean that when things need to be faced head on and dealt with assertively, that there is an underlying element of fear of change? The forthright and outspoken character may find that added frustration creeps up as they 'say it how it is' during times of challenging behaviour from the patient. Demands for extra help and support may be made when sadly they are not always at hand.

On this road we tread it is like trying to get the scales to balance so that patience is around when needed and constructive assertiveness expressed when we need to.

No two people will grieve this journey quite the same. The most upsetting thing is to give yourself permission to grieve as a carer. You are doing the very best you can with the skills and talents God has endowed you with.

So what about the one diagnosed with Alzheimer's?

CHAPTER 6

Brian's Perspective

Brian by nature is a kind, considerate, gregarious gentleman with strong principles, and he sees this world very much from a 'black and white' perspective, e.g. *the punishment fits the crime*, or if someone has to go to prison for an alleged offence, that is, don't dig deeply into their psyche for a reason and help them recover. This means that, although he has an intuitive spiritual side, logic plays a major role in how he sees the world.

One can see how this has challenged his journey from diagnosis with Alzheimer's to now being in full time care. Prior to this whole journey, we would have interesting discussions, thankfully with a good sense of humour, where Sylvia would always be looking deeper into situations and want to see how the real 'God' deep within the offender could be resurrected and rehabilitated to make a positive contribution to society. Brian's *black and white* view could not be shifted. How did we get a balance? Sylvia would at some point say, "You know, darling, you are absolutely right with how you view the world, it's just that I view it differently

– and you know that is OK!" That one phrase valued him and allowed us both permission to stand by our own values together. Even now, as time has passed and his condition worsened, this Brian is still able to acknowledge the blessing in our relationship of neither individual seeking to control the other.

So how has Brian dealt with his journey with Alzheimer's? Prior to diagnosis, as others around him were observing changes in his general behaviour, he was 'carrying on regardless' and not seeing any differences in his routines. One example is associated with cutting the grass at the front and back of the house. Over the years he would have religiously kept both front and back regularly cut to perfection. Over time he did not seem to notice the grass grow. Sometimes he would receive a call from one of his customers that he had left his diary behind and a return journey would be made as if it was quite the natural thing to do, and not unusual for a man who was an absolute perfectionist with how he carried out his day-to-day business.

He would prepare for his barn dance events as usual and not be aware that some equipment was missing; to him he always had a great evening. The other band members did an amazing 'cover up' to ensure that the punters had a great time. I was always told what a great night they all had and how well it all went. Maybe in some ways it is a blessing for the patient to be oblivious to what is happening. Yet when life challenges become overtly apparent to those around, dealing with them is another issue. Denial plays a major role in the disease's progression. I know that Brian courageously admitted that he had some problems when I sat down with him to suggest a GP check up. He also showed great outward courage on the diagnostic journey, and would say, "Well I just have to go through this, don't I?"

On the day of diagnosis he allowed outward emotion to show by his absolute silence on the journey to the hospital. Once in the consultant's room his nervousness showed in his facial expression and body language. When he was told that he had Young Onset Alzheimer's Disease his typical 80% logical character said, "It's not what I wanted to hear, but I will live with it as best I can." On the way home in the car, he said, "Well, I don't feel any different and I am healthy, so I'll get on with life."

Over time he has talked about how he wished he could turn the clock back. Frequently he has asked me with a puzzled look, "Why can't I do this?" Doing up his trouser belt, for example. "I've been doing it for years?" He would transpose frustration with a task to the equipment e.g. trying to get the petrol mower to start, "F*****g thing! It's always started first time before!" One day at least three years after formal diagnosis, we were sitting at the dining room table after our evening meal and he began to talk about how he hated not being able to do the things he used to do.

Suddenly he began to sob uncontrollably as he released all the inner pain of his diagnosis. "It's awful not being able to drive, I loved my car. Barn dances were my life and now it's all gone!" As I hugged him and allowed him to let it all out he blurted out, "Sometimes I wonder if it is worth going on, if it wasn't for you and all you do for me!" Without being patronising I told him how good it was that he released all the deep emotions and that we would carry on the journey together and be as positive as possible and enjoy our time together. It was as if this were his final acknowledgement of the journey he was on at that moment. It has been enlightening to witness his perception of what is going on through a brain with very compromised neurones.

We would go somewhere for a dray trip or on our final holiday together for a week in a caravan. Sylvia would be doing her very best to deal with 24/7 'naughty neurones' and have grumbles wherever we went. However, at the end of the trip he would have a happy smile on his face and say with great gusto, "Well, that was really lovely. I really enjoyed myself!" I did not reply with an angry outburst – instead with a smile and a twinkle in my eye, I would add, "We did have a few naughty neurones but I am glad that you have had a good time (inner thoughts, mission accomplished!)."

As I write this story of our journey, Brian is now in full time care in an excellent care home that specialises in dementia and Alzheimer's. Puzzled at first as to why he had to stay a while, he accepted the need for sleep assessment – he was typically a nocturnal patient five to six nights a week. He has settled well and gets on well with the staff and most of the other residents, and joins in activities. Night time continues to be a challenge, but he is pleased to see me when I visit and has not yet forgotten who I am or the love we share. He does on occasion have a minor naughty neurone manifestation, but with staff around it is more easily dealt with. He has certainly adjusted to his new home, while Sylvia is dealing with her own emotions around the new routine.

He will say how he misses me when I visit, and his perception of time being affected makes him say, "Where have you been? You haven't been in to see me for ages!" A quick reminder that I visit every other day mostly and have Sunday lunch with him will usually help reassure him. He enjoys it when we go on a minibus trip together and shows a happy, smiling disposition throughout. My goal is to facilitate him being able to positively express himself with me as long as possible in whatever way his neurones allow.

I have been in awe of how he has dealt with this journey thus far and am living as Eckhart Tolle (writer and speaker) would say, 'In the moment.' One thing is for sure, the Alzheimer's journey is a great teacher of learning to be in this moment and do one's very best to be at peace, no matter what is going on around you.

In spite of angry outbursts from Brian as he was

adjusting to the inevitable journey of accepting help with day-to-day tasks like personal care and getting dressed, he gradually adjusted to changing routines that were subtly introduced and became less angry, he would even find humour in the changes from time-to-time.

How those times of his barn dancing band days are a great memory to both of us. I recall a Saturday evening when I would dress myself in black trousers, red shirt and specially purchased black shoes and socks and go to Brian's home, where he was methodically loading the heavy band gear into his car. From speakers to amplifier, guitar and other sundries – recorder and tambourine along with carefully chosen dances to suit the audience. Novices would have a very basic set of dances, and those who were regular annual clients were teased with more complicated dances during the evening. Everything was packed into the car in order of required setting up procedure and carefully protected with blankets from the garage shelves.

Excited at the thought of participating in the evening with the man I loved and his friendly band crew, I jumped into the passenger seat and off we drove. Occasionally, I would be navigator from a printed map – no Sat. Nav. or GPS in the earlier days! On arrival we are greeted by the other band members and Sylvia watched as they set up the equipment, and a light box with their illuminated logo. StockBroker Belt, very appropriate for a Surrey based band, I always thought! Instruments all in tune and break time confirmed with the organiser, the fun begins.

"Ok, folks," Brian calls, "let's have long ways sets of six couples with ladies facing away from the door and the men facing the door." Very clear instructions, but we watch as there are some confused faces as to where 'facing the door' is and 'facing away from the door' is. Time for Sylvia to go to the rescue and get six couples sets in line. The band start up the introduction and everyone is in full swing to "Go in 2, 3, 4, and out 2, 3, 4 and cross over and face your partner." This is repeated and the instructions continue with men walking round the ladies and the ladies walking around the men, and the top couple galloping down to the bottom to make a new top couple.

There is much laughter as some forget it's time to "Walk round the men and women," and then they get out of rhythm to the music. So what! They get it in the end and at least are having a great time.

More dances, with Brian and I demonstrating steps and moves, and we have a well-earned break and are allowed to indulge in the splendid cuisine created by the organisers. Brian with his big appetite piles his plate with meats and salad and rolls, much to the embarrassment of the other band members. My plate is decorated with few items due to my wheat and dairy intolerance. Never mind. I have my trusty cool bag with me, healthy salad and dairy free yoghurt. Oh how

I would love to indulge in the black forest gateaux that seems to stare at me saying, 'Eat me!' Of course, Brian can fill up on a grand mix of all the desserts!

Break over, the entertainment continues, and those not driving are beefy men and more 'merry' and unable to tell left from right or make a simple square shape of couples. Sylvia comes to the rescue again and somehow manages to sort out the mess. At least they are having fun. We both loved being able to join in some of the dances, with comments like, "Oh dear, we have got the experts with us! Better get it right," or "Oh, we have the experts, that's great!"

By the end of the evening we are all tired, but with a wonderful sense of achievement from helping others have a fun evening, whether it had been a birthday party, wedding, annual reunion or a charity function. We still recall those wonderful times, and Brian says he would love to put the clock back. Truly I am blessed with the most precious memories as his journey progresses.

Some years before Brian showed signs of his Alzheimer's disease, he was a real local radio fan and regularly called the programmes, becoming well known to some of the presenters. He also visited the studio from time to time, which he thoroughly enjoyed. Before his deterioration requiring full time care, I became involved in the local RadioWoking.co.uk internet radio station. Having been interviewed about my published autobiography, *From there to Here – Journey of a Skinned*

Rabbit, the show invited me to co-host once a week, and trained me up to a standard of being able to present my own show. Brian would come to the studio each week and sit in on the show, really enjoying being in the atmosphere and meeting many of the guests. He so loved this whole experience, and Roy Allaway, my co-host, would tease him in a friendly way, and say, "OK, Brian, you're our security man." Which Brian loved. I also got pleasure from him being there with me.

CHAPTER 7

Finding the Blessings?

With the Alzheimer's journey being such a challenge, you may ask how one can find any blessings or, as Sylvia would say, 'divine gifts' in this journey. Life is a journey of experiences designed to help us find that inner part of us that I believe is the spirit or 'God self' and bring that through into our day-to-day life.

It is through tremendous challenge that we can find the inner strength we never thought we had; we can learn how to find and journey towards the light at the end of the tunnel.

My nursing background saw many patients and families having to deal with terminal illness, death and grief. I watched couples who seemed to grow closer together as they coped with terminal cancer and other chronic diseases. Yes, some seemed to become withdrawn with a lack of communication, and both parties playing 'pretend' games thinking the other person did not know about the diagnosis. Those who acted out denial games had the greatest emotional trauma: those who were open and honest, with support and counselling, became strong and found positive moments along the way, living life to the fullest for as long as possible. True, Alzheimer's is a very different ballgame, as it were, and probably one of the most challenging diseases to cope with because of how it manifests itself over time.

Yet I can honestly say that our journey has brought us closer together as a couple, and during the earlier stages, gave us a determination to make the most of every moment without creating a 'claustrophobic' relationship.

For many years we had lived separately and spent time together between homes, and we had a good balance of quality time and space to do those things that were part of our own working and private lives. We both felt a need to have some degree of independence, even though there was a deep love between us. Maybe past experiences meant that we were both carrying a fear of full commitment to some extent, who knows? Once Brian was showing signs of Alzheimer's, we spent more and more time together – much of it at my house. It was as if he felt a subconscious sense of security as I gradually took the lead in day-to-day life.

We had always talked things through over the years, and that became one of the great blessings on our journey. It allowed Brian to express his feelings, and our love for each other deepened. I know that I definitely wanted to support him right through this journey as if I were his wife. I cannot count how many times during the early to mid stages that I was thanked for all I was doing to help him. He became more spontaneous in sharing his love and wanting to take me out for meals so I didn't have to cook. We frequented our local Harvester restaurant and, as his cognitive skills began to show signs of deterioration, the waitresses were very good at supplying extra napkins to protect the table from the spillage from his overloaded salad bowl. Our last visit was for his birthday in February 2014, which he thoroughly enjoyed, leaving me with very happy memories.

The Christmas after he was diagnosed we spent at Brian's home together. It was very special and he was very relaxed. I could see that he felt under no pressure, and we spent lazy days watching DVDs and going for walks where there were many dogs he could meet and make a fuss of.

Early the following January I noticed a card addressed to me lying on the dining table, and when I opened it there was a 'Thank You' card from Brian for giving him a lovely Christmas and New Year. I still have it in the office upstairs. It brought tears to my eyes and reinforced my determination to stand by him no matter what. We have come to appreciate miracles in what might be seen as the small things in life. Just a coffee and cake in a garden centre together was a joy, any trip to illustrate as much independence for him as possible. I learned to accept and see the pleasure he got from his 'helping' me by cutting the grass and tidying the garden. Challenged with the lawnmower, I would have to take over and watch as he would pull up a few blades of grass meticulously from the edge of the grass and put it in the garden bin. He felt he was doing something useful, and I would thank him and say how much better the garden looked. To see him fulfilled was a blessing for me.

On this journey we travel we need to appreciate even the smallest of things the patient achieves, much like a child.

I have certainly seen a more sensitive man develop over time, and his verbalising needs emphasising of how much he loves me has made this sensitive woman cry many times. One of the most joyous moments was to see Brian realising more and more that he wanted Sylvia to fully be a part of his life. His need for more support threw us together where we cohabited every night and spent more time together in the day. Rather than being a burden, we became even closer, and then the day dawned on Valentine's day of 2013. Brian went to his coffee club near his home and I went to pick him up at the usual time. As I walked in he stood up, looked at me straight in the eye and said, "You're late!" Slight pause. "But I will forgive you because you are going to marry me, aren't you?" Although we had discussed whether it would work, and I had said a while back, "If you *ask* me to marry you, I would," I was not anticipating a proposal!

Shocked at the proposal in front of so many people, I was speechless for once. Then one of the ladies blurted out, "Sylvia, you are going to say yes, aren't you?" Reality immediately sank in as I said, "Of course I will!" Loud applause from all ensued, and we left as one very happy couple, with the diagnosis seemingly irrelevant – only deep love and togetherness was important.

Planning our wedding was a great diversion from the day-to-day challenges, and Brian seemed to show energy I haven't seen for some time.

We decided to get married on 1st May, which would have been my mother's birthday, and we were delighted when the Registry Office were able to confirm that day. The Registrar was very supportive when we had the booking meeting and she communicated with Brian in a way that was legally acceptable but that enabled him to feel the minimum embarrassment, because of his inability to read properly due to the posterior visual cortex atrophy. Honesty with his diagnosis facilitated understanding and helpfulness, for which we both were very grateful. I had, however, never doubted the success of booking the wedding and, as would be my usual practice, put the situation in the hands of God and the angels.

To see the happiness radiating from Brian's eyes as we began our preparations for the day gave me a wonderful feeling. I felt blessed to have this man in my life, not only to be the wife he never thought he would find after a bitter experience years ago, but to journey with him during any future challenges on the path we were travelling.

Over the years we have been together, talking things out prevented major rows. In spite of all the 'naughty neurone' incidents faced in the last couple of years, the wonderful memories I have of the real Brian remain deep inside as a wonderful expression of our divine selves sharing earthly experiences. No, Sylvia is not living in the past, she is rekindling past experiences to help deal with current challenges. The more we focus on the joyous times we have had in life, the more we can be helped to overcome our current challenges. The inner joy can then be felt even in the darkest moments and wash away grief and pain. How I value the sensitivity that has developed in my man through his diagnosis. How wonderful it is to have the moments we share when he expresses his love for me, which seems to come from deep within his soul.

I am *TRULY BLESSED!*

CHAPTER 8

Suddenly the Rocks on the Road Appear

Yes – the road following our decision to marry suddenly became an extremely rocky ride. My father used to talk about 'The Rocky Road to Dublin,' and here we were about to experience the rocky road to marriage! Although well and truly behind us, I vividly recall the day I had a phone call to say that the marriage could not take place as someone had put a legal caveat on our wedding. 'A Caveat,' I thought, 'whatever is that?' In all my years of nursing experience I have never come across that one!

The shock we felt is indescribable, it was as if someone had stabbed our hearts. The first thing Sylvia did was look on the internet to find out what a caveat was. After a search I found the information on a government website. Apparently if anyone feels that a wedding should not take place for any reason they believe, for the sum of twenty pounds (£20) in UK currency they can fill in a form and send it to the registrar. The couple planning to marry have to provide evidence to show that – in Brian's case – he has sufficient mental capacity to decide to marry. Shock turned to understandable anger and, for me, a determination to ensure our wedding would go ahead. Thankfully, I am gifted with determination in a crisis – my nursing background!

Within days we had gathered what we believed was sufficient evidence to ensure the wedding would go ahead, and even the registry officer was amazed at the results. We breathed a sigh of relief and continued plans for the wedding. I decided to make the wedding cake as there were dietary challenges to consider – Sylvia being wheat and dairy intolerant and Brian having to avoid alcohol due to his medication restrictions. Also, if a member of my family should attend who is allergic to eggs..?

I have made many cakes over the years and am blessed with talent passed on from my mother. I did delegate the icing of the cake to a friend as she was up to date with these skills and I was rather rusty. The last major project, including icing, was for a married couple in my nursing home who were celebrating their diamond wedding anniversary, the chef with speciality cake skills was away on his holidays!

Recipes were adapted and cakes successfully baked and passed to a friend to ice for us. We had decided to keep our costs to the minimum – even my lovely pink sapphire engagement ring was secondhand, as I felt I wanted to wear a ring that perhaps had a sad story to it. There followed a search for a bargain wedding dress. Luckily in our town there is a bridal outlet where they sell sample dresses at amazingly good prices, and I got a really good deal. It did need altering, but another blessing appeared; my dear friend, who was to be my matron of honour, was an excellent seamstress and offered to do the alterations for me, saving around a hundred pounds.

Things seemed to be coming together and we felt confident that the wedding would go ahead on 1st May as originally planned. Oh my! Another 'rock in the road' appeared. We were called to a meeting at the registry office and there were further developments to the caveat. A request had been made for Brian to have a medical assessment to prove his mental capacity to get married, which meant we would be advised to have a solicitor to help us. Brian agreed as he felt he had nothing to lose. Time was now ticking by, with little hope remaining for a May wedding. The impact on Brian was beginning to show, and he became depressed as well as angry. I was concerned as to how this whole saga would impact on his Alzheimer's, as stress was the last thing he needed at this time. To see his joy of marrying me now being questioned was heartbreaking, and we took off one Friday to my friend and Matron of Honour to be, to have a break and some sea air. Brian had had an assessment by now with the help of our solicitor, and things were looking good for the wedding to go ahead as planned. But then yet another 'rock in the road' – the assessment had been questioned by the party who had put on the caveat, so the wedding would not take place. I vividly recall this moment: we were in our friend's car and my mobile rang. It was a call to say yet again the wedding was not able to go ahead. I froze and couldn't stop myself from sobbing with grief. Brian too, sitting in the back of the car, was distressed and shocked. We immediately went back to the house and sat Brian down in a chair – his colour had changed to an awful grey, and showed signs of intense panic. My friend was about to ring for an ambulance as Brian said he had pains in his chest. He was administered rescue remedy, which is a great natural remedy for stress, and a cup of tea. Gradually the colour seeped back into his face and he showed no further signs of any physical damage to his health. We did get him checked over by the GP on our return home, and there were no signs of any major impact on him. Our solicitor was contacted and he got to work on a strategy to deal with the situation that had arisen. It was now beginning to look like the 1st May wedding date would not happen. Inside my faith was strong, and I knew that something would turn things around in our favour. Our hopes were raised by the strategy that had been devised that would still enable the wedding to go ahead as planned. Sighs of relief!

Sadly our hopes were shattered once more over what seemed minor issues, despite solicitor input, and 1st May for a wedding was no more – leaving everything in the hands of our extremely capable solicitor once again.

We had planned a few days away in a caravan from 3rd May as a sort of honeymoon, which we decided to continue with as a short respite from all the turmoil. In beautiful parkland with lakes, the caravan was like a wonderful retreat and we relaxed and began to enjoy our privacy. We knew against all odds we still had each other and our deep love for one another. Then another blow came – a phone call from the registry office to say that there was insufficient evidence to allow the wedding to be rebooked. This time the shock of the call overcame both of us and even my faith was tested to the limit. I retched with an acute tummy upset and Brian too seemed poorly. We took a trip into the local town and, as I am a great advocate of the holistic approach to shock and trauma, we looked for a health food store. With no-one else in the store I explained our situation to the lady owner. She immediately grabbed a couple of herbal extracts, gave a dose there and then and advised on the dosage over the next few days. What an angel she was!

Exhausted, we drove back to the caravan and did our best to keep our spirits up, using some good old-fashioned prayers and invoking Archangels Michael and Raphael for healing and protection from the negative energies coming at us. The next day sadly I was not fit to drive, so we spent the day relaxing in the caravan together.

The drive back home on the final day required inner strength and involved much angel assistance, as well as frequent stops for us to relax a while.

When we returned home a conversation with the solicitor gave us hope, as he had a final strategy. Brian agreed to yet another independent assessment with an eminent Psychiatrist, who was also well versed in legal matters.

By now I had my friend on standby with the cakes, carefully monitoring their condition. She had iced and decorated ready for 1st May as we had expected. In spite of her frequently checking the cakes, we learned one fateful day that because there was no alcohol in the cakes – only fruit juice – they had fermented and were no good. Back to the drawing board, Sylvia. The saviour of the wedding cake was Brian's trip for a routine assessment. He had now been transferred from the original consultant to the mental health department, and so we attended the appointment in June as previously arranged. The usual questions were carried out and general discussion with us both. The consultant, when discussing Brian's medication stated that as far as she was concerned a small amount of alcohol would not do Brian any harm. Wow! He was overjoyed after nearly four years without even a Gin & Tonic. I have to say here, though, he did say that he had not really missed the alcohol and was not desperate to get 'drinking' again.

However, Sylvia now had her solution for the wedding cake – by adding alcohol to the replacement cake it should keep preserved until we overcame all the challenges and achieved our desires.

Back to the assessment, and something very interesting to note in respect of the impact of all of the trauma and distress around getting married. In January of that year his scoring out of 30 was barely into a moderate score at 19.5. In June of the same year his appointment rendered his score to be 10 out of 30! My feelings are therefore that on this journey, to aid a slower deterioration, we need to minimise as far as possible any extra stress on the patient.

In spite of this, when Brian attended his two hour in-depth assessment with the psychiatrist, the outcome was wonderful! *He had proved categorically that he had mental capacity required not only for marriage but other important legal matters!*

With this report in the very capable hands of our solicitor, we knew that things would turn out in our favour. With over forty years of family law behind him, a successful outcome was at last reached on our behalf. There was so much love and support during this difficult time, and so many prayers were being said on our behalf. Somehow we managed to keep a strong faith deep within us as we rode the waves of the storm.

The reasons for sharing in quite a lot of detail our experiences are twofold:

1. We need to be aware of the potential on this early journey for others to see situations quite differently from those in the thick of things, and be ready to deal with any challenges that may arise. Ensuring any legal protections that are necessary are in place is also essential.
2. If one can stay in touch with the higher self within, and stay united in the desire and goal, faith and determination grows stronger and an overcoming spirit rises up.

What was very interesting, and a joy to witness, was the improvement in his score six months after we were married, when he was happy and relaxed. In December it had risen to 15 out of 30.

Both Brian and myself have acknowledged how the challenges we went through did indeed make us stronger, and we know the importance of standing in one's true power – the inner power of the spirit self. This is the power that draws to us solutions through people that manifest in front of us as we 'let go and let God.'

I illustrate this before ending this part of our journey by sharing how we came to have such an amazing lawyer. Sylvia was attending a business networking meeting as part of the holistic coaching marketing, and in among a room full of various entrepreneurs, she just happened (or not!) to get talking to our lawyer's wife/secretary and take a business card. There was something about her whole energetic presence that struck me, and the way she explained how their independent practice worked. When we needed a lawyer I somehow knew I should call them. For me this was definitely synchronicity, or a 'divine incidence.' I do not believe in coincidence, but do strongly believe in 'God incidence.' It has served me for many years, and even brought about my meeting the man who was to bring me the love and relationship that was perfect for me.

We truly *are* soul mates.

So what happens next?

CHAPTER 9

Yes You Can!

It was a Friday morning in the July of 2013 and, as usual, I was up and around at 7 a.m. Brian was still sleeping and I went downstairs to carry out my morning yoga and meditation. I had just got to the bottom of the stairs when my mobile rang. Whoever is this calling so early, I thought? The display showed the solicitor's name, so with baited breath I answered the call.

"I am sorry to call you so early," he said, "but I thought that you might like to know you can now get married." I rushed upstairs. "Wake up, Brian, and take this call," I cried with joy – when he heard the same words I have never seen him so wide awake at 7a.m. "Get up," I said excitedly, "we have to get things organised quickly. We must get to the registry office as soon as it's open and book the earliest date." My mind was racing – phone friend – Matron of Honour. How soon can she and her man be free? An early text to her, "Are you up?" Then a phone call and before 9 a.m. we had confirmed the days they could be available.

As calmly as possible I encouraged Brian to get

dressed while I did breakfast – I didn't want him to get flustered – mind you, his excitement over being, at last, able to marry his lovely lady, overcame any chance of being flustered!

By 9.15 a.m. we had made it to the registry office and crossed our fingers for a gap during the next week – preferably Wednesday or Thursday. Almost a miracle, their diary showed a slot at 2.30 p.m. on Wednesday. What a wonderful July that we at last were going to see our desire fulfilled.

There were the final plans to rush through in four days, including the Saturday and Sunday! Hairdressers, makeup, afternoon tea at a beautiful hotel close to the registry office with both the bride and Matron of Honour gluten free! This had better not be a challenge.

In amongst the last minute dash to get everything in place we decided it would also be nice to have a church blessing at our local spiritual church. That was to be about a month later to fit in with the minister, who would take the service; that gave us just over four weeks to pull it together. Somehow the relief of the wedding actually happening seemed to calm Brian down and he was in good spirits.

The hotel agreed to do gluten free food for us, which was a great relief. I did emphasise gluten free cakes as well – fresh fruit, although healthy, was not an option on my wedding day!

My dear friend's partner agreed to do the

photographs for us on both days, and an album was to be their wedding gift to us. We felt genuinely blessed after all we had been through. Even my makeup was to be a gift from another friend, with natural and healthy products. Brian, having been in business, had a perfect suit and tie for the occasion without extra expenditure. All that was required was a new white shirt – not a problem with all the major outlets close to where we live. He had not put on a tie for some years, and I was concerned that it might challenge him, but I knew that my friend's partner would help here without flustering him. From friends and family we had excitedly notified, cards began to arrive. Oh, we were so excited beyond words! In amongst the excitement I made sure that everything was done as calmly as possible and without panic over the few days we had.

I was 'crossing everything' that my wedding dress would fit, as weight had dropped off due to stress, even after the alterations had been completed.

The day was very soon upon us and I got up extra early to allow for Brian to be calm and able to take time with his washing and dressing.

Off to the hairdresser for creative styling for a bride and groom. Brian's cut and blow dry was slightly different to the usual, but he liked it and looked really handsome. Well, more handsome than he always had! It was his looks and smart classic dress that was the initial attraction.

Back home and then the makeup girls arrived, and we did a take-over for the kitchen so that Brian was not left totally alone. He was amazingly calm as well as nervous and excited. We reassured him that he would be absolutely fine answering the questions for our vows – the registrar had made them simple and easy to understand so that Brian only had to say "I do," as "Yes" will not suffice – it is not legally allowed as ceremony language, so we learned. Counting on some of the 'quality' neurones, we frequently went over the vows to help him. He was very good about this, although I will never know how humiliating for him it must have been facing up to dealing with just being able to say "I do."

Just as my makeup was finished there was a ring on the doorbell – Shirley and her partner had arrived. Wow! We would be driving off to be married in his brand new bright red Jaguar, which was festooned with blue and ivory ribbons to tone in with the theme of ivory and sapphire blue. Shirley and I left Brian to chat with her partner and he kindly assisted with his tie as well.

Upstairs we started getting into our wedding gowns – me first with bated breath. I stepped into my wedding dress and was zipped up at the back by Shirley. I had lost weight! Now this is where Brian's obsessive saving of things just in case they are needed came in very useful. On the windowsill was an old lightbulb cardboard box jam packed full of safety pins. My Saviour! Deftly and with patience I am pinned together and fitted into the wedding dress.

Now it's Shirley's turn – we hold our breath again as she has been attending slimming world. Yes, you have guessed it. Here come the safety pins again! How many I had in my dress I cannot recall, but I do know I used at least 12 to get a final 'Matron of Honour' profile!

Time is now fast ticking by, and we have the challenge of getting Brian into the car at the front and preventing him from seeing me at the back. I also need to get downstairs with great care in my securely pinned dress, complete with quite a long train at the rear!

I am both excited and nervous for both myself and Brian – I so want this to go off without a hitch. I am successfully 'arranged' in the back of the car with Shirley, and off we drive to the registry office.

Next challenge? Get Brian out of the car and into the registry office without him seeing anything of me. Shirley's partner did a sterling job of this, keeping Brian distracted till I entered. Then there was the emotional moment as the bride greets her husband to be and sees the loving look and great surprise at my wedding gown. The registrars usher us into an anteroom to go through the service and check a few personal details. Thankfully, Brian could recall the answers even after all the stress of the caveat and its effects on his memory a month before our wedding. Brian expressed his nervousness at dealing with the vows and was reassured by the registrar: "Don't worry, Brian – the last couple I just married had none of your challenges and I had to go over the vows I do not know how many times!" I saw him visibly relax and we prepared to walk into the lovely room overlooking the gardens with the sun streaming in – it was a wonderful warm, sunny day with a clear blue sky. God was definitely shining on us on this special day. I had tears in my eyes as Brian responded to the vows with absolute perfection. I was so proud of him.

His challenge with signing his name had been quite a problem over the last year or so, and he was unable to sign in a straight line. Again, they were amazingly understanding and, thankfully, our entry was at the bottom of the page and could allow for his downward scrawl.

When the words "I now pronounce you man and wife. You may kiss the bride," were uttered we were both overcome with emotion. At last we were what we had wished to be, and would treasure this day forever – and so we have... but more of that later!

The only other people present on this day were our lawyer, his wife and granddaughter, who was with them on that day. After all his hard work he deserved to witness the event. With the sun pouring down and blue skies above, photos were a must in the gardens, before going for our afternoon tea.

We said goodbye to our lawyer and his wife and

granddaughter, and drove a few hundred yards up the road to the beautiful hotel for a bridal afternoon tea. On arrival we were greeted by our personal waiter and escorted to a private alcove that was already set with a variety of sandwiches, including a selection in gluten free bread. An old-fashioned cake stand was bedecked with cakes, *but* I could see that they were all full of wheat and dairy. Alongside was a large bowl of strawberries. Yes, they looked delicious, but on my wedding day there was no way I was not going to indulge myself in cakes. I exercised my right as the bride and called the waiter over. "Where are the gluten free cakes I ordered?" I asked.

"Ah, well!" was the slightly embarrassed response. "The chef did try to make some gluten free scones, but they did not turn out very well."

'Update chef training then!' I thought to myself as I responded with, "This is my wedding day, I requested gluten free cakes. The strawberries look lovely, but we would like some cakes."

The waiter went a bit red and replied, "Just a minute, I will talk to the chef," and he scurried off. A couple of minutes later he returned to say, "I have had a bit of an argument with the chef and told him what we want. Give us around 20 minutes please." Next we were plied with extra free Champagne! When he said he'd had an argument with the chef, I said to the others, "Never mind an argument, I have worked with chefs in the care home when I was matron! Chef probably went crazy and shouted uncontrollably to the poor waiter, who was only trying to please the beautiful bride and her friends."

Surely enough, in around twenty minutes another cake stand arrived with a variety of cakes and some warm scones. I said nothing, but it was obvious that someone had been sent urgently to the health shop in town to purchase cakes and scones, which were then warmed up! Luckily for them they had a good choice of cakes. Now we have to eat them all! Brian and Shirley's partner, who had good appetites, helped us out. Of course, we did eat the strawberries as well! Why not?

We were presented with a box by Shirley and her partner and inside were two beautiful silver goblets and a bottle of Champagne – this just rounded the day off wonderfully.

In spite of the dilemma, all did go well and we looked back later together at what was a perfect day with a deep sense of joy and relief. Brian was also very tired and needed nurturing during the evening. Fortunately there were no 'naughty neurone' episodes. No time to relax though, the church blessing is only a few weeks away!

CHAPTER 10

Get me to the Church on Time!

So now the challenge is to organise the church blessing with all speed whilst keeping life as calm as possible for Brian. In the excitement of being able to have our union spiritually blessed, it could be so easy to create situations where Brian would become agitated and show those typically angry traits as a result of frustrations, as Sylvia was quickly getting things organised for the day.

In amongst all the wedding preparations I had finally given up my own house and moved into his, cramming clothes etc. into whatever space I could find in a house that was full of 'we may just need that' items – including clothes he had not worn in years! I was subtly creating space without him being aware. Interestingly, in spite of his Alzheimer's symptoms he would know if something had been moved, so careful negotiation was required so that things were still seemingly in the same place. It was challenging trying to incorporate my personal things in his house full of a lot of unnecessary clutter – of course, to him it certainly was not that. It was very important to balance adding my touches to the house while allowing

Brian to feel he was fully maintaining control of his life. He dearly loved me, wanted me with him as well as appreciated my help, but at the same time, he did not want familiarity around him disrupted.

I frequently reminded him how much I loved him and how happy I was to be his wife and to provide support where needed, and that seemed to keep a calm atmosphere. Thankfully, at this stage of the disease Brian was sleeping well and only needed minimal assistance with personal care, such as getting his clothes out in the morning. He was still able to wash and dress himself successfully. I suspect the twenty-four hour presence of his wife had a subconsciously reassuring impact on him. He was more relaxed, knowing that he didn't have to cope on his own. He was now coming out to the kitchen quite often with tears welling up in his eyes as he hugged me and thanked me for all that I was doing for him. He would say, "I really don't know what I would do without you." These moments helped greatly as I could see it genuinely came from his soul and made up for the times his disease manifested itself with angry outbursts.

The church preparations went fairly smoothly and our good friend and minister came to see us regarding how the service would be conducted and to discuss hymn choices with us. Again, Brian was reassured as to what he would have to say, and because vows had already been sealed lawfully, Sylvia would be the main responder. This was a great relief to him as he wanted to 'do it right.' The patience our dear friend and others showed at the church was very moving. We would do a practice run of the service routine after services to reassure Brian that he would be fine on the day. There was quite an array of what I call 'God influence' over music to be played as we processed from the altar to the back of the church at the end of the service. Brian and I had discussed using one of his favourite songs, but we couldn't come to any decision on this.

We were dying to get another run through of the music with the organist and as we finished confirming the hymn tunes, he suddenly began to play a tune that was one of Brian's favourite barn dance tunes played by his own band. "That's it!" we both excitedly cried out – his face alive with joy. Brian added, "Why don't we do a Polka down the aisle?"

"What a great idea," I tentatively replied. A thought did go through my mind then, Polka = Glory as to Brian keeping in step if he doesn't quite get it right – me in high-heeled wedding shoes, plus dealing with the long train on my dress – like everything else in life, I knew I would pull it off! Of most importance was to make sure that the day was full of joy and that he had a really great time. Who knows how long I have with him at this stage of his journey?

A typical ceremony aisle was speedily created and a practice Polka carried out with all the folks still mingling over their tea and coffee clearing away. Brian was in his element as he led me down the aisle at full speed! "I think we need to go a little slower," I suggested. I will have a wedding dress to cope with and my high-heeled shoes and, after a few goes at it, we got the rhythm and dance speed perfect and Brian travelled home a very happy and excited man. Thanks to internet design and print and Sylvia's creativity, we were able to speedily get out invitations to family and friends, using email and the phone to confirm. The order of service leaflet was easily generated online thanks to Microsoft Publisher and Vista Print. I was gaining Brownie Points, as we say in the UK, for achieving all that was required on a strict budget. The print service leaflet would be divided between church and home with family returning to the house.

Now continues the saga of the wedding cake. The final decision was to have one iced fruit cake and cupcakes. The cake had to be egg-free to accommodate one of my nieces, and the cup cakes gluten free with a vegan diet also taken into account. A local cupcake coffee shop owner came up trumps here with gluten free and vegan varieties – all at a good price too! More Brownie Points for Sylvia! All seemed to be going really smoothly with the preparations, and I had reassured Brian that those coming back to the house would have plenty of space to sit – many times over of course due to memory problems. How grateful one is for a patient personality, so necessary on the Alzheimer's journey. Then – two days before the day, Sylvia made a *huge* mistake: Brian decides that we must cut the grass in front of the house and make it look really pristine and tidy. Not a problem, you may say! Hmmm – Brian and grass cutting is now a challenge. In his head he can do it, and this is his chance to shine as my husband. What actually happens is this. Brian says he will cut the grass. Sylvia in her wonderfully thoughtful way suggests we get someone to help him as he has challenges with the lawnmower. Oh dear! "I am quite capable of cutting the grass! I have been doing it for years!" he retorts.

"But darling," I respond gently "– you do have challenges because of your posterior cortex atrophy."

"What? Do you think I am f*****g stupid or something? That's it – I am not coming on Saturday. It's off! Or you can go on your own!" I have triggered major naughty neurones. He takes himself to bed and is adamant that he will not be attending the ceremony on Saturday. Still learning how to deal with outbursts, I am now distraught and in tears (not good in hindsight). I know I must leave him and quickly get dressed, grab my mobile phone and tell him I am going out for a walk.

"That's OK, you do what you like. I am not going to the wedding!"

Trying desperately to hold myself together, I walk to our lake and find a seat. A call to my dear friend and Matron of Honour calms me as I am reprimanded lovingly about how I dealt with the situation whilst I release with tears.

After a few minutes of panic, peace returns and I nervously return home. Brian is still in bed and I leave him – after a while I make breakfast without mentioning the grass cutting. Eventually he calms down and the front garden was left as it was – not looking too bad at all really. 'Why did I not just let him struggle with the grass and subtly help him?' I thought to myself during the day. I had completely destroyed his confidence and sense of male pride in doing his bit towards our day. This journey is so unpredictable and we are continually adapting in each moment. Balancing caring and helping with facilitating the patient's own sense of independence is like walking on a tightrope at times.

By Friday morning we are 100% back on track and making final preparations for the next day. Not a word was said about the grass cutting and Brian didn't mention it either. To prevent any undue stress on the day, I decided to have my hair done the evening before and do a final touch up on the Saturday. Thank goodness for an amazing Hungarian lady who did my hair for a very good price, and who was creative as well. Extra hairspray was applied to 'glue' it in place. To prevent agitation with Brian, I made sure that the Saturday morning routine was securely in my head and on paper as he was concerned about 'timings' etc.

He was in good spirits on rising with understandable

nerves about getting it right during the service. I secretly sent a text to our neighbour, who has two lovely dogs that Brian adores and regularly visited. My request was a visit during the celebrations at home after the service, so Dennis the Chihuahua was on standby for later.

I involved Brian as much as possible in arranging the furniture, so that he felt needed and happy. We had visited the church on Friday evening for a final rehearsal – floral display, and celebration drink delivered – non-alcoholic purely because of Brian's medication and those who were driving.

Once again we had a beautiful warm sunny day, so the outdoor table and chairs were set out on the patio. Brian seemed relaxed and was looking forward to seeing family members on both sides. His gregarious spirit was rising up just as before his diagnosis.

Before we could blink, the morning had passed; Brian was dressed in his wedding gear again, minus tie, which he would be helped with on Shirley and partner's arrival. They arrived on cue with the decorated red Jaguar as before, and Shirley and myself went upstairs to get changed. It was now the moment of truth with our wedding gowns – will I need safety pins or has the weight I needed piled on for me? Joy of joys, the dress fitted perfectly! Shirley's needed a little attention due to her ongoing slimming classes, but thankfully I had not hidden away the safety pins. This time the happy bride and groom sat together in the back of the car feeling so happy, though nervous. I asked the angels to help us through the celebrations and with our Polka down the aisle. The joy of being with family and friends without any of the pre-wedding uncertainties was wonderful and the Cancerian bride was indeed feeling exceedingly emotional. Brian was the proud husband and looked contented, happy and yes, so handsome!

He was able to follow the entry instructions well, and went through the service with perfection. It was as if God and the angels were giving us a really special memory to hold close to our hearts.

There were a couple of humorous moments. We had chosen four hymns, one for the start of the service, one after the vows and one before the start of the address by the minister and one at the end. As we approached the final hymn – and I had not noticed this, the minister, who had obviously had her own nerves about the service, announced, "Ooops! We haven't had the second hymn. Oh well – we'll just have to sing two together." That caused a laugh throughout. The organist was probably puzzled!

So the end of the service and the organist strikes up the Polka. The proud and happy husband grabs his bride, who just about gets control of her wedding dress, and off we go as the congregation clap to the beat. Not content with going from the front to the back of the church, he gets carried away with the music and starts to go back down the front again. Family and friends who were just leaving their seats to follow us just managed to clear the aisle as we sped up to the altar and then back again! It was good to see him having such a great time. Cupcakes and sparkling wine to toast the couple followed, and Brian was in his element chatting to everyone. You would not have known that he had Alzheimer's in these moments. Even Sylvia was able to relax and fully enjoy the moments with him.

After the photographs friends dispersed and family came back home with us. I was ordered out of the kitchen by my two nieces as I went to turn on the oven for the potato bites. "Out of the kitchen Sylvia! Go and be a bride with your husband!"

Dutifully I obeyed and joined Brian on the sofa. A little later, as we are in full celebratory flow, the doorbell rings and there is little Dennis – nickname 'Dennis the Menace,' as he rules the other dog and cats at home, standing to his full 'height' and ready to take on the audience. Brian's face lit up even more as his little friend pranced into the living room. He looked around at everyone as if to say, "Who will I go to next for a fuss?" Suddenly he was centre stage at the event, and we even had photographs taken of him sitting on my lap, which finalises the photograph album prints.

Sadly the day moves on and family, Matron of Honour and partner have to leave, but oh what a day to remember! We have recalled our wedding days many, many times since, and this is our favourite memory that

Brian still retains. Unfortunately, due to his accelerating posterior cortex atrophy, he cannot fully recognise the photographs, so I talk him through the days instead and enjoy the visual memories for myself. That aside, we have been blessed to be able to have very, very special memories to recall. Brian was very tired after the day, but the joy of it all seemed to compensate and the evening went without a hitch: we both went to bed a very happy couple.

CHAPTER 11

A Scary Honeymoon

The intended few days away in May as a 'honeymoon' went out of the window due to the major upheaval to the wedding. A very good friend of ours who lives in Lincolnshire offered for us to go and stay with her for five days, which we both agreed would be a lovely relaxing break after the trauma we had experienced. As a qualified nurse and a quiet and outwardly calm person, I knew that she would be a support for me with Brian and his challenges. For example we were going to what would now be unfamiliar territory to him, as it had been at least a couple of years since a previous visit, which I remember very well! It was a short time before Brian's driving licence was taken away, and to say I was glad to get off the A1 and arrive in Stamford is an understatement. He was driving too close to cars in front, not judging slowing down and his stopping judgement was a nightmare. St. Christopher, patron saint of travel, and the angels were called upon all the way by me. He did let me drive part of the way home, thankfully, after a near miss with a car coming the other way in the dark. On the post-wedding trip, Angela did the driving whenever we went out thank goodness.

So Sunday morning after our lovely wedding service is spent preparing for our trip to Lincolnshire. Brian was encouraged to help with the packing and I patiently reassured him that everything was packed apart from personal care and food items. I say patiently because I lost count of how many times he asked me throughout the rest of the day. Ugh! Those 'so and so' memory neurones, bless him.

With the weather still warm, we set off on Monday morning complete with a snack and flask for a short stop en route. Brian was in good spirits, but he also slept part of the journey as the excitement of the wedding blessing day was still being felt. He was so different from the pre-diagnosis man who had loads of energy and could stay up late and then go to bed, head on pillow, and be asleep in less than a minute. But of course, one of the symptoms of Alzheimer's is intermittent tiredness, probably due to the neurones that are synapsing extra hard.

The 'natural break' and snack stop went smoothly and Brian performed his now obsessional routine of prolonged hand-washing after handling food. A napkin wipe just will not do!

We arrived safely in Stamford and were met at the car for help with luggage and assistance for Brian with steps up to the pavement. His posterior cortex issues were now making any stairs other than familiar ones a challenge.

A well deserved cup of herbal tea for Sylvia and coffee for Brain was served, and we light-heartedly asked if he could remember previous visits. For me it was lovely to be with someone who is very 'instinctive,' and who goes about things slowly and calmly, along with having the physical support for a few days.

A trip into town triggered memories for Brian and he was relaxed and happy – especially with a large cappuccino to indulge in whilst out and about.

Back at the house we stayed and chatted and one would not have known that my lovely husband had any challenges. They did of course manifest overnight with negotiating the bathroom and successfully managing pre-bed routine tasks. Once in bed he slept all night, thankfully. Next morning washing and dressing went without a hitch and the stairs were coped with successfully. With breakfast and health-giving supplements all ready for us, it was like being in a friendly guest house.

With the weather warm and sunny, a day trip was the plan, with Angela as driver and guide. Knowing Brian's love of animals, we took a ride to an animal sanctuary with sheep, goats and farming memorabilia. Having purchased our supply of food for the sheep and goats, we set off on our 'animal trail.' Brian was in his element, feeding the sheep and goats, laughing most of the time. I still have a video memory of this day to cheer me when I return from the care home; it saddens me at how he is now compared to that day.

Stamford in Lincolnshire is home to the famous Burleigh House where the Burleigh Horse Trials are held each year. HRH Princess Anne was a regular competitor in her youth. A visit would not be complete without visiting. Brian, still in good spirits, was up for it. Our timing was perfect – the day before the horse trials were due to commence. We were able to walk around the exhibitor area and view a variety of horsey memorabilia and men at work. We kept this part of the visit fairly short to accommodate Brian's visual challenges, and as his concentration span was relatively short, I did not wish to trigger an 'agitator' incident and have him getting angry. Photographs were a must under one of the trees that was at least six hundred years old.

Careful negotiation of the rope boundaries in place and we made our way through the gardens to the refreshment room in the great house. Tea and cakes went down a treat, cappuccino for my man, of course. A walk around the fish pond filled with carp of various colours, and then we made our way back to the car as Brian was tired.

On this trip Brian still had the ability to co-ordinate his eating skills and, if we were out, he was able to independently go to the toilet without losing his way coming back out. Oh yes – this happened quite regularly not long after our honeymoon. It was no good Sylvia being shy and retiring. I got used to looking for a gentleman who I felt would go in and rescue him without it being obvious.

If a security man or the owner were around, they too would be asked to help out. I have always found that if you ask for help, people really are kind, helpful and patient.

We visited the beautiful Lincolnshire Cathedral and enjoyed the calm and uplifting energy in the building. I guided us to a small chapel within the cathedral and lit a candle. We sat in the stillness for a few minutes, eyes closed. I felt I must give thanks for our time together and Brian's love, as well as asking for the angels, Jesus and God to help me on the future journey together. In spite of the Alzheimer's disease I knew I was blessed with his unconditional love.

On our return home we both felt refreshed and happy – life gradually got into a routine, where I combined caring for Brian with my holistic coaching services.

CHAPTER 12

Life is Somewhat Settled

The joy of actually being married remains uppermost in our day-to-day life and we begin to make minor adjustments around the house without destroying its familiarity for Brian. He was beginning to need more prompting with personal care and help with choosing clothes, and I was noticing him struggling with shoelaces and getting jumpers and coats to be 'compliant.' If I tried to help, his frustration would turn to a mild outburst of anger, so with patience I allowed him to struggle and eventually get things right. We would now have a coat flung down in anger at times and shoes thrown across the room as he struggled with the laces – no, we definitely were not going to change to slip on shoes, they were not macho!

In spite of his needing more help, I could leave him for two to three hours safely at home listening to the radio with a drink at hand. Sometimes he drank it, sometimes not. We would go for bus rides on a Saturday and have lunch out – a simple meal such as ham, egg and chips that Brian could manage easily. When he was in really good spirits and wanting to express his gratitude for all I was doing, we went to our local Harvester and, as usual, adorned the table with our paper napkins to trap the salad overflow; and the main course would be grilled salmon fillet with chips and peas for ease of management! I recall the first visit some months previously after our visit to the mental health consultant, when he was told a little alcohol would not harm him. Always liking a typically English ale, he ordered a pint. As soon as he tasted it his face contorted; "Well, isn't that odd? Because I haven't had any alcohol for so long, I really hate the taste of this!" Thinking on my feet, I suggested we change it to a bitter shandy. That went down a treat, with facial contortions turning to smiles.

We had by this stage been attending posterior cortex atrophy support meetings and had been alerted to the power of using bright colours, especially red, as contrasting to other colours to aid recognition. Following their suggestion, and with Brian's co-operation, I called the Sight for Surrey Team, who are linked to the Royal National Institute for the Blind. A lovely lady came to visit and we were told that in our town there were two other people with the same diagnosis of P.C.A. Poor Brian had to go through a questionnaire aided by myself due to his many issues. The outcome was the loan of a speaker clock to which she placed red tape around the top and got Brian to press the black button in the middle. Hey presto! We had the time of day announced. It took a few practices for him to successfully recognise the square box and find the button, and I was unsure how successful it would be.

We also had a return visit bringing a telephone that had large numbers on it. She placed red tape onto the receiver and Brian was able to successfully lift it and return it to the base. Red tape was also applied to a button and marked with a big letter S in case he needed to call me when I was out. The reason for this was that when I was out, I always called him to make sure he was all right, or I would be on my way home. The normal telephone challenged him and he had difficulty putting the receiver back onto the telephone base. If he had tried to take a call when I was out, sometimes the receiver was not placed back properly. Of course, Sylvia then phoned and got the 'engaged' tone.

Even with the special phone we did begin to have challenges with Brian's time-clock, so I decided to reduce my networking meetings and focus on online activity around his care. We were both happier and did more things together, and the outbursts were kept to a minimum. He seemed to have plateaued, and on our next mental health assessment his score had gone up by 5 points to 15 – not surprising as he was now married, settled and happy.

Before we knew it, Christmas seemed to be looming. Brian asked that we spend it at home together quietly, relaxing and watching some films, and I was happy with that idea. As we were now on a diet to supply extra nutrients to the brain, as well as planning wheat and dairy free festive fare, I decided I would go right back to basics and make everything myself, swapping fats for coconut oil. Thankfully I love cooking and would produce really tasty meals that were simple and healthy that he enjoyed. I had always been grateful for having a man who loved food and would eat anything – except strong garlic! Very useful when I am wheat and dairy intolerant. Brian watched and enjoyed reminiscing with me over the great cooks our mothers were, and there was much jollity and laughing in the kitchen as I prepared homemade mincemeat substituted with coconut oil as well as the Christmas pudding and Christmas cake. I even made an alternative filling for sausage rolls using soya mince, as we were not lovers of pork.

Before the festive season we would usually visit one of my nieces and her family in Wales. This year, older sister was visiting from Scotland for Christmas and we were invited for a weekend stay. The family was four children, now aged 20, 18, 16 and 15. Their mother – my niece – was a schoolteacher and used to working with children with challenges. The way the children had been raised meant that they understood Brian's challenges and were amazing with him.

We arrived on the Friday and were shown to our own room, which had an en suite toilet and shower.

Thankfully the main bathroom was only a few paces down the landing for bath time and personal care. Brian was also sleeping well at night now, thanks to a mild night sedation. He was really happy to see everyone, and they him as well. Being a large family, there was a good sized downstairs toilet, and I would regularly assist him when he needed to go. Understandably he did get very confused and disorientated with which direction to go to the large kitchen/diner and conservatory lounge. With lots of help on hand I could relax and have a break from my full time caring role.

When we went shopping on arrival, I did need to remind my niece to take it slowly so as not to leave Brian in one of the aisles when he had a 'blank' moment. She was like Sylvia – clear the aisles, I am here to get the shopping done. I had over time slowed my walking pace to almost a stop, otherwise I would regularly lose Brian in the supermarket. His excuse for a blank moment was that he was browsing and looking! By now I was rehearsed in a quick look behind to make sure he was with me. Did people around think I had a nervous twitch as I frequently looked around? I have found myself doing it if out with a friend who is walking behind me due to people getting in the way! Mealtimes in Wales went pretty well – I warned my niece we used napkins at home to catch spills. She subtly put out paper serviettes on the table and everyone used one so that Brian didn't feel different from the rest of us.

We had fun looking back with Brian on our visit when the children were small and the games he used to play with them. A favourite memory was a Christmas when we played 'hunt the thimble' for hours and watched as the eldest girl kept finding it and the younger ones cried out, "It's not fair mummy, I never get a turn to find it!" The eldest was duly told to let them all have a go at finding it. Brian had been so good with children over the years. They loved him like a close uncle and both my nieces always said he was the uncle they had never had. When I remind Brian he always has tears in his eyes as he remembers.

By Christmas I was 100% focused on caring for Brian and doing my best to motivate him, which was challenging as he always had a relatively boxed in life that he enjoyed, i.e. sales representative in the kitchen industry for years, folk singer, barn dance band organiser caller, plus his spiritual mediumship work. He was not an avid reader, even though the house was littered with books of all shapes, sizes and subjects. He had never had a television, and I had actually dispensed with mine a few years earlier by begrudging a licence fee I never used. So we would watch programmes on 'catch up' – a regular was Songs of Praise on Sundays and we would sing along. I also looked for music concerts on YouTube of favourite singers such as Daniel O'Donnell and other folk/country singers. Music really got him in good spirits.

A typical day by this time went like this. Sylvia gets up around 7 a.m. and goes downstairs to spend time doing yoga and meditating, to connect to her higher self and start the day from a state of inner peace. Brian would be in bed still quite sleepy. Breakfast is then prepared and Brian aroused to start his morning personal care, with assistance from me. He came down and had his usual porridge with coconut oil, MCT oil and molasses and a cup of coffee, along with essential supplements of vitamin C, omega oil and vitamin B complex to feed the nervous system. Breakfast completed, we returned upstairs to get dressed while he did his 'toilet' routine and washing. Shaving was assisted, as was dressing, but allowing him as much independence as possible, which would include a few choice words as underpants seemed to somehow get back to front initially after I passed them to him ready to step into! Socks too often went on the wrong way round.

By the time the routine was completed and I managed to do my own hair and makeup, we would be downstairs by at least 10 a.m. and he was ready to just 'sit' on the sofa. BBC 2 resounded around the house, his favourite morning radio and dependent on discussion topics his mood and topics of conversation would flit between humorous to Alzheimer's anger outbursts. I took him out for a coffee most days to distract and prevent any naughty neurones kicking in. I had learned over time that boredom will easily precipitate confused thoughts or hallucinations, and generate outbursts that needed gentle approaches. Evenings were about finding something that entertained on the laptop or local radio. A must to listen to was the Paul Miller Show on Radio Surrey at 10 p.m. and attempt at the quizzes. This finished at 11 p.m. when the bedtime routine kicked in. By the time I eventually tucked down to sleep it was at least midnight, but it was important to maintain his routine.

He was still sleepy at night thankfully right up to and after Christmas. He enjoyed sitting with me as I wrote Christmas cards and we reminisced over the old friends he had still kept in touch with. I had no idea this was to be our last Christmas together at home as we prepared for our quiet time together. We attended a carol service at our local church, and I could not help but remember the time in earlier days when the Aricept side effects were causing fainting attacks. He passed out at the 2011 carol service and we had called an ambulance. We managed to get him to the back of the church – we were sitting in the second row! He picked a great time too, as the person taking the serve was leading us in a meditation healing invocation. With great calm and sensitivity she invoked specific healing to Brian. It was beautiful. The evening did end with some humour after Brian had been checked over and was deemed fit to come home. We offered the ambulance team tea and mince pies. Laughingly I said to them, "I bet this is the first time you have attended a spiritualist church – but don't worry, nothing spooky happens here!" They had a good laugh and I am sure had a good tale to tell colleagues back at the station. This carol service was enjoyable and went without a hitch, as Brian was now well and truly fixed with his pacemaker.

Our wish for a peaceful Christmas came to pass and Christmastime was a delight. We had wonderful closeness without any naughty neurones rearing their angry heads.

2014 was to be a very different year with a taste of it in New Year's Eve 2013. We were in the kitchen and Brian was trying to communicate something to me and, as was beginning to happen, I struggled to fully understand and respond correctly to what was in his head that he was trying to say. I used this phrase as communication is a major challenge. Suddenly he had a strange look in his eyes, his facial expression changed and verbal abuse came out: "What's up with you? Are you f****** stupid or what?"

I took a deep breath and tried to calm him, but it did not work. Unfortunately he was in the doorway, and I couldn't escape to give him space. Another tirade of abuse was uttered as he punched me in the abdomen. It hurt a bit, but I knew no damage had been done – a dose of Bach Flower Rescue Remedy helped when I could get to it. He moved and I was able to free myself, walk away and put music on, which in time distracted him and brought back the Brian that was still present most of the time. While it was all happening I was internally invoking peace plus Archangel Michael to protect me. This always helps bring a calmness beneath any human element of fear. It is so important we give off as calm an energy as possible during these outbursts. Boy, was I to need my Mantra, "I choose Peace," whilst invoking the angels in 2014!

CHAPTER 13

Oh my! What is Happening Now? The Blue Badge Scenario

So we are beginning a year that should bring us total happiness now we've been married for around six months. It was not to be.

Brian was generally relaxed and happy to be married at last, but still expressing a lot of anger at what we went through to actually get to our wedding. I had mixed emotions over the whole saga of pre-wedding events. There was the natural human anger, but also a deep sense of sorrow and a feeling for the need to forgive and ask for healing for those involved. We hoped that they would also learn from the pain that had been caused to both them and us. Forgiveness did not mean I was pleased with what had been done, but I was not willing to carry resentment and anger towards those responsible for delaying our happy event.

Fortunately our deep love was giving us joy most of the time, and communication around the Alzheimer's situation was still positive between us early in the year.

It was during my morning meditation one day in

January of 2014 that I heard a voice saying "Something will happen that will trigger respite for Brian." I did not panic nor was afraid, I just acknowledged it and continued in the stillness prior to calling Brian for breakfast. Interestingly, after this message was given to me, events began to take a sudden turn and would never go back.

Suddenly Brian began to present 'sundowning' symptoms:

- Wide awake at bedtime and ready to chat for a long time.
- Confusion as the evening progressed, even with the lighting kept bright as recommended.
- Hallucinating when we got into bed with added confusion.

Along with the sundowning symptoms he began to be generally more confused and unable to concentrate for long periods. His personal care routine was changing rapidly with much more input from myself in the morning, at bedtime and with going to the toilet. I was also becoming increasingly aware that his posterior cortex atrophy seemed to exacerbate things.

Following advice from the Sight for Surrey visitor, Brian agreed that we should apply for a blue badge. This was to be another very interesting journey. By now I am familiar with how best to fill in government forms and, with the aid of our Sight for Surrey key worker, the paperwork was duly completed and posted, along with those dreadful looking passport photographs they like these days – the 'when was he let out of prison' look! In a few weeks we had a phone call that was *almost* amusing.

A lady's voice on the phone said, "I've got your blue badge form here and need to make an appointment for Brian to have as assessment." I should add that this is at the time of the major flooding in the winter of 2014 in the UK, and we live in an area where towns within 7 – 10 miles of us were very badly affected as a result of the river Thames bursting its banks.

I knew some kind of assessment would be necessary, but was not quite ready for what I heard next: "Brian needs to have a physiotherapy assessment to see how far he can walk." 'What?' I thought, 'he has Alzheimer's, not a physical disability!'

My response was, "There is nothing wrong with his legs, so if that is the type of assessment he will surely fail."

Then the strangest reply came. "Oh! What a shame! I am doing a clinic in Woking this coming Saturday as Staines is still flooded and I need to fill my clinic!" I certainly was not going to waste our time 'filling her clinic' and declined the offer fairly curtly.

The next course of action was to call the P.C.A. support nurse, who immediately drafted a letter and created a blue badge protocol for those with posterior cortex atrophy, which I received by email before the end of the day. She was to be our saviour. I was not giving in, I never have in life and was not going to now. Time to help get changes for Alzheimer's and P.C.A. sufferers. Just because the patient can still walk does not mean they are safe when getting in and out of the car or in judging distances. By now, Brian was a bit of a nightmare getting in and out of the car, and making sure he was with me as we negotiated the car parks. Holding hands as a happy couple was a suggestion on how to cope with this, but he always refused.

Within ten days we had a letter stating that we'd need Brian to be assessed by a nurse at the Staines Clinic – the floods had abated and all that was left was dirty roads and piles of sandbags.

With bated breath we arranged an appointment, successfully negotiated the roads and made the clinic with time to spare, and for himself to get bored with waiting! We were called by the nurse, whose room is at the end of the corridor, and of course Brian strides down in a straight line and negotiates the doorway with no problem! We sat down and the nurse was an absolute angel. I joked about having been a district nurse and we had an immediate rapport. "Those forms are stupid!" she said. "They just don't fit your husband's criteria." There followed a couple of poignant questions and a few scribblings on our form. "That should do it. You'll get the badge in a couple of weeks." Relieved, we left to go home via a coffee shop to celebrate with a cappuccino and a decaffeinated soya latte.

Sure enough, in two weeks we had our blue badge. Then there was 'icing on the cake' – we could apply to our local council for a 'proximity card.' This is a posh name for a special card in a protective plastic sleeve that allows you to scan car park entrances and exits anywhere in the borough to obtain free parking. That was completed overnight so I could breathe a big sigh of relief about trips out. Even Brian soon forgot we were in a disabled zone and enjoyed the extra space, and of course the free parking.

All that was left to deal with was ensuring he was with me at all times, and not suddenly lagging behind with the potential for me to leave him, which frequently happened in supermarkets. However careful I was, at least he wore a distinctive colour coat or jacket so I could easily identify him from a distance! If we travelled further afield at least in the parking area we had made up for having to pay. I did make one early mistake regarding this: I parked in the appropriate bay and took Brian for a walkabout and coffee, but returned to the car to see a yellow and black plastic bag on the windscreen – yes, I had been fined! Lesson learned – always check the parking charges board.

Talking with some other couples at an Alzheimer's Society lunch subsequent to our blue badge success, we learned that one lady had given up appealing on their application and was putting up with enormous rows with her husband in the local supermarket's car park because of challenges negotiating around cars to get to the entrance. I assured her that with patience she would succeed and that it was essential we made a stand for Alzheimer's sufferers and their right to benefits, to give as good an experience in life as possible.

I must also say that, whilst taking action at a physical level and being terribly practical, I combine this with visualisation and invoking the help of angels as well as blessing the mail or email sent: yes, it does help!

CHAPTER 14

We Did Have Clear Cut Goals!

At the beginning of 2014 we still had quite clear goals in mind for Brian's Alzheimer's care. This was our plan:

- Keep care at home for as long as possible and aim to see it completely through at home.
- Have home care as symptoms progressed so that Sylvia could still combine Brian's care and support with her other divine purpose activities.
- With home care, have a carer/carers who would be committed for the long term to create stability for Brian. This would mean Sylvia could have breaks with confidence in the continuing care and trust someone being in the house.

Whoops! A great dream that unfortunately could not realistically be lived out.

Following his outburst on New Year's Eve, Brian began to show further changes in respect of general life skills and was requiring more of my time. I was now not leaving him in the house alone as the Crossroads Care visitors were so busy that we were still on the waiting list. Brian was also reluctant to have 'strangers' in the house and believed he was OK.

Every day was about doing my best to keep Brian stimulated and be on my guard, as he was very quick to become angry and have quite aggressive outbursts. All this after virtually no sleep at night and a massive invoking of the angels for help and regular meditating 'I choose peace.' Friends were amazed at how well I coped, but that is who Sylvia is. We may have a crisis, but we come through it and then just get on with life.

The first major incident of early 2014 was when Brian became angry and abusive after I said something. He was stamping around the living room with the typical Alzheimer's angry look in his eyes, which means I have to just be calm and keep out of the way. He stormed angrily from one end of the lounge to the other and grabbed half of the long drop heavy curtains. I watched nervously, allowed him to calm down and quietly picked up the curtain and draped it over an armchair. He was completely oblivious to this. It was evening, so I decided to go to bed and hoped for a good night. As I recall he slept quite well, probably exhausted with the outburst.

Next morning I was apprehensive about how I explained the lack of a curtain at the window. Over breakfast I just said that his naughty neurones had kicked in and made him angry, which he seemed to accept. Our good friend and cleaner was due that day and, on arrival, had the sense not to say anything, but with my help quietly put the curtain back. Everything was intact and just needed rehanging with a little bending of part of the track. Brian sat and watched without a word and remained calm. Phew, was I relieved!

I was still holding my weekly spiritual meditation group at the house, which Brian loved, but he was just drifting off somewhere during the evening. Luckily they were friends and understood. To suddenly stop this would have caused yet another outburst.

As the year progressed towards March, we were both frustrated about what was happening and, after many chats together in his more rational moments, we agreed to try and get a full review of things.

I called the mental health team and looked into day care once or twice a week at the local Alzheimer's day care centre. The mental health team arranged an earlier review and I heaved a sigh of relief when Brian – albeit reluctantly – decided to try day care following a meeting with the day care manager. For him this would have been a very difficult time as he was seeing himself progress on the 'awful' journey.

The day dawned for his trial run and, my-oh-my, what a morning that was. Extreme anger about it and refusing to go, but I managed to get him in the car and to the day centre, where he continued his bad mood. After lunch I went to bring him home, but his dark mood was still around and he refused to go ever again.

I hid my upset and tried diversional therapy, taking him for a cappuccino in a local garden centre. Gradually he began to calm down and I reassured him that I would not take him to day care again.

I talked out with him the idea of a review, and also considered applying for a higher rate of mobility allowance now we had a blue badge. More money being involved generated his compliance with this one. We had help with this from a volunteer who worked with the Woking Hub Centre. She was a lovely lady, herself disabled who showed up with her dog in tow. That was all we needed to keep Brian calm about how we had to answer questions focusing on really bad days, as he would keep saying, "But I can do that!" or "I don't need help with that!" Feeling confident, I posted the form and waited. The usual 'We are considering your application' arrived. Hopes began to rise for a positive outcome *until* another letter arrives – 'We have considered your application and Mr. Stock is not eligible for extra mobility allowance, but will retain his high care rate.' We could of course appeal, which we decided to consider following a review.

By now we are into May and I had booked an appointment with the GP to register the situation from my perspective and give weight to a review form for the increase in mobility rate. Now let me backtrack here and remind you of the 'inner voice' in January that said something would trigger respite. Well, the doctor's visit was to be *very* interesting. I walked into his surgery, sat down and began telling the story of our journey, and that I wanted it noted that although I was coping, there was stress involved. "Let me check your blood pressure," he said. I had reported all the sleepless nights I was having. "Hm…that is very high!"

"Don't tell me," I retorted.

"Well, just say it's around 200/110." Hastily he writes out a prescription with the advice, "Get this prescription now and take a tablet, then one a day, and come back on Friday" (it was Tuesday). The words I had heard in January echoed in my head and I knew I needed a rest to recover my own strength and regain some sleep.

I talked to Brian and added to what the doctor said that it was essential I had a rest to eliminate the risk of strokes. He agreed to go and see the manager of the local Princess Christian Care Home, where we had previously met the manager. "Anything to help things," he said, and hugged me, and we both had tears in our eyes. I called the care home and the manager was able to see us. A very emotional interview ensued with Sylvia tearfully explaining the situation, and a very caring manager getting Brian's agreement to have a week of respite care. This was to turn out to be a 10-day stay as the GP requested there was a 24-hour blood pressure monitoring and I wanted to really feel rested at the end of the respite time.

The emotions I went through as we packed clothes

and other things were intensely upsetting at having to put Brian into a care home so soon after we had been happily married, along with a sense of relief that I was going to have a break. Brian was very quiet as he was understandably worried about his wife, but also somewhere within himself challenged at having to go into a care home.

Brian was now having coconut oil and M.C.T. oil (Medium Chain Tryplyceride) daily, along with other key antioxidants and brain supplements. These were also sent with him and, from my own experience, I typed a detailed routine to assist the carers and nurses in achieving the very best care for him. I included information about his past love of running his barn dance band and folk singing, plus the challenges of posterior cortex atrophy. We admitted him on the Friday afternoon and I agreed to stay away for 2 – 3 days to really be rested. That was hard to do as, although I was relieved to have 'me time' to recoup my energies, I so wanted to see him. I knew that we would now have to begin day care and that the journey was taking a new turn.

This was now a time when I would more and more begin to draw on my inner 'higher self' strength and work through the emotions of guilt and sorrow at what was happening. Yes, I had put behind me to a great extent the whole marriage caveat scenario, but I could not help thinking that the stress and trauma of that whole episode had impacted on his progression. Then of course oneself talks and says that ultimately it is all part of the earthly journey and all is in divine order. I was beginning to feel that I needed to take council with the Dalai Lama as I was desperately trying to walk this path from my Spiritual self as a coach and teacher. My blood pressure rapidly reduced, the 24-hour monitoring showed a good average, and I was requested to continue the medication and return in six months time.

Brian seemed to settle well during his time in the care home and the staff were a delightful team. By the time he was due to come home, I felt stronger and rested and ready for whatever was to come.

Suddenly I became aware that it was coming up to one year following our beautiful wedding. Hm! How do we celebrate without creating the naughty neurone attacks? Tentatively I suggested to Brian that I should cook an anniversary meal at home, so we both dressed in our wedding clothes for the meal to create a special evening. I planned a simple but tasty menu with sparkling wine; careful timing and kitchen negotiations are required so that I can deftly serve dinner in my wedding gown with its long train! All goes well without any hitches, and Brian goes to bed a very happy and contented husband, and I have a great memory to log. During the evening we discussed having a holiday, and I felt it would be good to have at least one more together – well, well!

CHAPTER 15

A Holiday – Well Sort of!

Since Brian has been diagnosed with Young Onset Alzheimer's Disease Y.O.A.D., holidays have been totally different. With added challenges from his P.C.A. (posterior cortex atrophy), it was important that as much familiarity could be maintained as possible.

The break we took together that stands out in my mind was in 2013 – the caravan break that would have been a mini honeymoon! By now I was the full time driver, packer, preparer and trips organiser. Past nursing and business skills came in very useful here. Booking a holiday online was easy and Brian was used to my regular online activity with shopping etc. The caravan park was located in a woodland park with lakes in the county of Kent, not a great distance from historic Rye and Hastings.

Our caravan was a gold star plus, which had extra width, was very spacious, had its own parking space and was away from noisy children and pets. Ideal for someone who is hypersensitive to noise. All went fairly smoothly so long as I steered Brian in the right direction for the toilet and bedroom, as well as alerting him to where important things like washables and his razor were. The greatest challenge he had was taking a shower, and on the first morning the fun began. Insistent that he could manage, he steps into the shower, turns the water on and then realises that he needs to adjust the height of the shower hose. Oh my! There was this naked man shouting and swearing as he desperately tried to carry out this simple task. In seconds the whole shower hosing and head had become dismantled, and water was spurting everywhere.

"I did not do anything wrong!" he angrily shouted through the glass, with bits of shower tubing in his hands. I was fully dressed by now, but disrobed so that I could safely get him out of the shower unit, piece everything back together and help him start again. What he called the shower is best not written down, but suffice to say it was enriched with typical A.D. expletives! The shower was put back together and, holding my breath, I helped him back to have a shower. Success this time. Apart from this hiccup and the pre-wedding issues discussed earlier, the caravan break was reasonably manageable.

Not so the next holiday trip.

We had just enjoyed our post-wedding Christmas and I wanted to take him away for at least one more holiday. He was keen to go abroad, so I figured that I could manage a self-catering holiday in Malta, as they speak English and Arriva buses have bought out the old charabang company. My writing sabbatical also meant that I had familiarised myself with basic bus routes and identified the perfect self-catering apartment with bus stops right outside and across the road. The local shop would supply my gluten and dairy free requirements, so no problem there either.

Excitedly I booked a good deal with Air Malta and the apartment and we renewed Brian's passport, thanks to the very helpful lady in the passport office in London who helped with getting a signature of sorts to stay in the designated box. Poor Brian was both embarrassed and exhausted by the end of it all. So all we needed to do now is invest in a very lightweight suitcase and plan packing and airport transport. Packing discussions were interesting, as Brian still believed he could manage, and that his years of holiday packing was still familiar. I decided to divert discussions and face the day of packing when it came and, of course, the repetition that would occur, requesting whether or not this or that was in the case. Joy and excitement seemed to override any thought of peripheral challenges. Subtly I organised special assistance at the airports, including with Air Malta who are not based in the UK. Eventually the UK airport got my message about the kind of help required, and that no he did not require a wheelchair! Airlines please wake up to A.D.: assistance is needed but it does not fall into wheelchair category. I could just imagine the issue that would have ensued if we had been greeted at the airport with a wheelchair. Don't even go there, Sylvia! The daily denials require the 'I choose peace' mantra, never mind dealing with an outburst at the airport and potential for security involvement!

Here we are now about 10 days away from our holiday to Malta in June of 2014 and on the Monday morning I am greeted with 'my leg is sore and hurting,' as he shows me his right leg. With my nurse's hat on again, I examine his calf and it feels hot and is a little inflamed on the inner side. A call to the local GP luckily justifies an emergency appointment, which finds that he has an infection in the main vein of his right leg. Antibiotics are diagnosed with a return appointment booked. On the Thursday evening at bedtime I notice a very marked reddening going up into this thigh. With antibiotics in his system I felt a further GP appointment in the morning would suffice. This visit showed an acute vein infection and that he needed an urgent blood test, as he was a candidate for what is known as a blood clot or deep vein thrombosis that could shoot off anywhere in the body. The antibiotics were immediately doubled and I knew that he needed professional monitoring and rest if we were to go away on holiday. To prevent hospital admission I talked to Brian about him going back to Princess Christian Care Home to be cared for and help heal the infection. We also had to face up to now not being able to fly to Malta. I told him that we would instead have a lovely caravan break as soon as it was possible.

He ended up staying in the care home for 26 days on a triple prescription for double antibiotics whilst he was recovering. I got agreement from him to wear support stockings to help with maintaining good circulation, with his legs being elevated at all times.

This is emphasising my life philosophy. Maybe the Malta trip was over-ambitious on my part. So I went ahead and booked another Gold Star Plus caravan in a Devon caravan park. Even this was very much a 'living on a knife edge' experience by the time he was prescribed his third lot of antibiotics. I know that a natural product called Silver Shield would help the antibiotics and speed recovery, but NHS protocol prevented it. Never mind…I had a plan for when he was able to come home.

It was Tuesday before the caravan trip was due to begin on the Friday and, although there was still inflammation, we agreed with the care home doctor that it was safe for him to go on a caravan trip. Now I immediately put my plan into action and with Brian's agreement gave him Silver Shield 5ml three times a day (it is totally safe and non-toxic). I also gave him probiotic capsules to return the bacteria to his digestive system that the antibiotics would have destroyed. They were packed with everything else for the seven-night break in Devon, along with the fish oils and antioxidants that were his standard supplement intake. Not forgetting the coconut oil and medium chain triglycerides that he now had daily to help with the Alzheimer's.

As packing is completed and the day dawns for the drive to Devon, I am relieved that we are not flying to Malta. He is not in good spirits and ready to throw a major naughty neurones any moment, and says he does not really want to go. I try to calm him as best as I can, pack up the car and get him into the front seat and belted in. This is when the "sort of holiday begins".

I am shielding rude comments the whole journey, and we are not even halfway to Devon from Woking in Surrey when he threatens to get out of the car and go home. I am also close to being hit by him due to naughty neurones temper! "I choose peace," and invoking Archangel Michael is even challenging as I am praying for the A303 services to appear. Would you believe it? We came to a major traffic queue for miles and it is not even full holiday season! Abuse about choosing to go to Devon with threats about going home continue as I work on my own inner peace, desperately dealing with the underlying fear I do not wish to show as I know *CALM* is the way to deal with outbursts. At least I have tools I can use to help me. Maybe I was on yet another learning curve? You are trying to cope with all this Sylvia and not wanting to recognise the sudden deterioration that is occurring! A stop for refreshments helped a little, but only with his naughty neurones. I was realising that the major infection has affected him as well, as the blood tests and revealed a positive result for a potential thrombosis. Was he experiencing some grains of clots that had shifted? I would never really know, but certainly the leg infection was exacerbating his Alzheimer's manifestation.

At last we arrive at our caravan and it is as expected – clean, spacious and Brian likes it. I chose the double bedroom that is close to the toilet for night-time purposes. Unpacking completed by 4.00 p.m. and as the sun is still shining, a decision is made to go and find the sea and café for refreshments. Still not in the best of moods, we drive to the local beach area and, joy of joys, there is an ice cream kiosk. A large cornet does the trick. A smile and calm character emerges at last. Feeling exhausted but relieved, I return with him to the caravan to relax before making supper – making sure he keeps his legs elevated as his right one is still very swollen. The television helps a little – what is he going to be interested in? Closely situated to the on site shop, a walk allows a gathering of information for 'trips out.' On with my best hat – plan the next day and subsequent days out whilst Brian indulged in television interspaced with moody comments to me. As the first evening progresses I am on edge again as the sundowning traits like it had begun to at home prior to the vein infection episode kick in. Unfamiliar territory created acute major nocturnal neurones, plus I had developed a cough and had to leave him in bed and use a spare pillow and quilt and one of the fitted sofas in the lounge area. As I tried to grab some sleep

I could hear chattering from the bedroom and then a naked apparition appeared, wondering where I was. The best solution was to tuck him down in the fitted sofa opposite mine in the lounge, and he eventually fell asleep. This was very much the nightly routine for the whole seven nights with one 'night of nights' but with an amazing blessing for myself.

It was midweek and after yet another interesting day – more of that in a moment – we begin the bedtime routine, intermixed with Naughty Neurone Syndrome, and get into bed. Suddenly there is a tirade of abuse from naughty neurone issuing forth and I dare not even move as I might get hit. I called upon the angels and Master Jesus and began my mantra, "I choose peace in this situation!" Suddenly the bedroom is filled with light and I am encased in a violet bubble of light and an incredible peace and joy fills my whole being. I can hear Brian in the background performing his Oscar winning performance of naughty neurones whilst I am in a protection of Divine Light and inner peace. From that moment on it was as if I now knew that all I believed in and taught was truly available to us all! That in our darkest moments we can feel peace protecting us from what is going on around us. That wonderful experience transformed my approach to the rest of the holiday and I had the strength to cope with days out, which were another eye opener to where we truly were on this journey of ours.

Boy, oh boy, did I need that peace as the week went on! I planned days out that I thought would be enjoyable for him, – like a visit to a donkey sanctuary where he would feed and fuss the lovely creatures. So we arrived at the sanctuary, thanks to iPhone GPS, and began to walk around after coffee – he had his usual cappuccino. It's great to be outside with large green paddocks, and to see so many rescued donkeys, all very friendly creatures, who are recovering due to cruel treatment from their previous owners. It was a really moving experience for me, an avid animal lover and anti-animal cruelty. Brian, on the other hand, was totally in his Alzheimer's neurones for the whole walk around, and refused to touch any of the donkeys. He just kept angrily repeating to me, "I don't know why you brought me to this place! I've never seen so much f*****g s**t!"

We then had to find a place where he could go through a ritual hand-washing exercise with sleeves (including coat sleeves) pulled up to the elbows, as he continued to mutter the expression of the day. Thankfully they also had a proper disabled toilet on site as we are now at a stage where we definitely go into the toilet together to assist. Tired from lack of sleep, and he too manifesting post infection and sundowning weariness, I drove back to the caravan via the coast and stopped to buy him an ice cream, as this seemed to be the one thing that gave a little respite from the naughty neurones.

Once back at base, we are both chilled and lie as

bookends on the sofas for a while. I wanted his feet elevated and rested a while anyway.

Another interesting day where an attempt to bring pleasure turned sour, was a visit to Powderham Castle, as Brian was really interested in history. I parked up and got him out of the car and paid our concessionary entrance fee. We were given a pass that allowed us to come and go as we pleased all day. I was just hoping we might please him with a guided tour and some lunch. Having convinced him that the tour guide was gifted with great oration skills and a great sense of humour, we began the walk through the entrance gate to join the queue for the next castle tour. Well – that was the plan. Suddenly a tirade of anger came forth, just like the previous day. "Why the f**k have you brought me here? These places are all the same! I'm not staying here any longer." Peace and angels invoked, in spite of the entrance fee paid, I decided it was best to steer him to the restaurant and buy a cappuccino. We are now calmed down a bit, but the angry mood persisted throughout the day and we were sundowning overnight. At least I was dealing with it more calmly and laughing to myself inside as a coping mechanism. Later in the afternoon, the calm ice cream was also obtained.

We did have one day where the mood was really quite good, and that was a trip to Brixham to include a fish and chip lunch with local fish, and mine without batter (oh, I wish I could!). They were very busy and impatience did get the better of Brian, so I spoke to the lady serving us and explained our situation. "I fully understand," she kindly responded, "I have a family member who has Alzheimer's. I will speed up your order for you now." Sure enough, a couple of minutes later our meal arrived with a smiling lady who flattered Brian and got him smiling. People are very kind and understand if we have the courage to speak out about our challenges. Yes, it is another part of acceptance Sylvia had learned along the way, as well as from her past experiences. I suppose that peace and calm can be created if we speak out and find some way of subtly communicating to them.

I had our trusty RADAR Key for disabled toilets with me and a little later, as the bladder called us, we located the disabled toilet not far from Brixham harbour. It is 3 p.m. by now and, would you believe it, locked! I found the local authority phone number on a parking information board and called them, only to be told, "Very sorry, madam, but all our disabled toilets are contracted out to a company!"

"Well," I responded with understandable anger, "that does not help our situation right at this minute. What are we to do?" The solution turned out to be a longish walk to a community/seafront entertainment and café centre. Thankfully the bladder held out and the toilet visit was followed by yet another daily dose of an ice cream. Part of me was wishing we were back home, whilst deep down I was pleased to be giving my husband a holiday he deserved.

The journey home was better than the outward one had been. A picnic lunch was prepared prior to leaving as the weather was good and, thankfully, it had been so all week we were away.

I planned to stop at around halfway at a Little Chef with outside seating, where we indulged in our picnic. A natural break and we were ready for the off! Oh, no, not quite – I espied a couple who were exercising their two labradors – one black and one cream. Brian was by now sitting in the car. I approached the wife and asked if Brian could fuss the dogs quietly. "Why, of course," she said, "this one – the cream one – is a pet therapy dog." She brought the dog to the car and I introduced her to Brian. The dog immediately sat down close to the car to allow Brian to fuss her. His face lit up as he caressed her and spoke to her owner. I was moved – and am as I write – to see how this beautiful creature could change the mood of my husband in seconds. I believe in 'God incidents' and not coincidences, and I firmly believe that it was the case on that day. From that moment on we had a great conversation for the rest of the journey. Now, wait for the grand finale on what was a week of learning and digging deep into my conscious self to deal with the challenges.

We had reached home and unloaded the car – I immediately did a typically English thing and put the kettle on for a drink. Brian came into the kitchen and hugged me as he stated with a big grin, "Well that was a lovely holiday, wasn't it?"

"I am glad you had a great time," I lovingly replied whilst inwardly thinking, *MISSION ACCOMPLISHED!*"

CHAPTER 16

A Change in Challenges – Letting Go?

Back from holiday and Brian's leg is thankfully looking free from inflammation – but I did feel it would be a good idea to have a follow up with the GP, as there was a lot of scarring up the vein site and ongoing leg swelling. He was satisfied that the leg was as good as it would ever be, and agreed in his continuing to wear support stockings. I added to that a daily dose of Silver Shield 5ml as a preventative measure. More about Silver Shield in another chapter.

Daily life ensued with sleepless nights and Sylvia dutifully taking her daily dose of Amlodipine 10mg for her blood pressure, alongside natural supplements for general health and wellbeing.

Brian had adapted well to the care home so we discussed his attending day care twice a week for stimulation and a break for me, as I was pretty much on a pattern of 24/7 care now, with two nights a week reasonable sleep if I was lucky. Much as I deeply love Brian, I know at this time he needed stimulation from others as I was challenged to get him interested in anything. Reluctantly, he went to day care for the first week and it was reported that he had a good time. The next week was a different story. Naughty neurones and long nights of sleeplessness were a regular feature now, and on this particular Monday morning he exhibited a major neurone attack on me, and was almost violent in his refusal to go to the care home. Tearfully, I called the Home and told them he was refusing to attend and apologised profusely. They understood as this happened with other patients as well. I managed to get compliance the following week and from then on, even if he left home in an angry state. What was interesting to observe was his total change of mood when he greeted the staff at the care home. He went from angry naughty neurones to responding to their welcome with, "Yes, I'm fine thank you – how are you? Nice to see you!" I would raise eyebrows subtly to the receptionist as I left. "You should have seen him earlier!"

When I went to pick him up I was told he had interacted well with people and enjoyed his day. I was usually told the opposite and, "I don't see why I need to go anyway. I'm perfectly OK!"

By the autumn I was really feeling the strain of caring and trying to create quality time with Brian rather than fielding the mood swings every 24 hours, so we had a chat with the mental health nurse during his October mental assessment visit. At this visit my notes were quite different as I wrote about angry outbursts both day and night. It was becoming a common practice now for me to leave him for a while at night and either go downstairs for a while or into a bed in the spare bedroom. Sometimes we both ended up downstairs having a drink and chatting over things as he came out of his naughty neurone phase. It was again heartbreaking to see his disbelief at his behaviour, even although I glossed over the whole scenario with, "Oh, those naughty neurones kicked in for a while and some choice words were said to me." It is painful enough for them on their journey without it being 'rubbed in' with detailed analysis of angry violent outbursts of which they have no recollection.

So it was agreed by all, including Brian, that we would have an assessment for help with personal care in the morning, as I was now providing assistance with all personal care needs. This was to be the catalyst for the next phase of the journey, which was not on my 'care goals' list. Twenty-four hour residential care.

It was the Sunday evening before his morning care would commence. I had made strong stipulations about time and on regular cover, as some of my past experience had been in agency community care and I know that carers were under pressure and did not always arrive when requested. Neither did the same carer always turn up, not good for Alzheimers patients where continuity and consistency is key to their positive management. The usual bedtime routine takes place and we do our usual goodnight routine and cuddle up together to go to sleep. Suddenly, on goes his bedside light and out of bed he jumps. I notice a typical 'neurones' look in his eye as we begin what is to be a night of nights I really don't want to recall. At the top of his voice he angrily and with expletives as usual but more vociferous this time, he throws the bedding off and starts throwing clothes and other things around the room. Quietly I pick up my iPhone, which by this stage never leaves me, grab a dressing gown, pyjamas, clothes and creep out of the room, as it is no use trying to calm him. He is like a wild animal. Doing my now commonplace peace invocation and working on being calm, I go into the spare bedroom and one of the beds. When I felt it safe, I crept out and turned on the main light in our bedroom and hoped it would trigger a diversion. No chance! So I left him, as he could come to no harm, and a few hours later I found him lying on the bed halfway down covered in the quilt. Nervously, I asked if he would like me to return to bed with him and got a gruff answer, "It's up to you – if you want to." Calmly and quietly I returned to bed, adjusting the pillows and quilt, but importantly, ignoring the mess in the room. I would deal with that in the morning.

Surprisingly, after agreeing not to have carers at home over breakfast, he was fairly compliant about going for day care that day. Making light of it, I jokingly told the receptionist after leaving him about the night's saga, not knowing it would be passed on to the manager with whom I now had a great rapport, due to my background and holistic coaching skills.

I spite of my deep spiritual self and the tools being used to cope on this journey, I was still somewhat 'on edge' in case he had one of his 'turns.' Thankfully the Monday night went reasonably well, apart from the now commonplace sundowning. However, his condition seemed to have really deteriorated since the leg vein issue. How different life was since the early marriage days – not that I would have changed anything, as our love was still as strong and I know the 'real Brian' loved and appreciated me. Most of all, now I had a desire to see our journey help others travelling the same road. You see, life is not all 'roses,' it is experience, and we are challenged to face it and find an inner self that has the courage and strength to help us carry on. Also, life teaches us in some circumstances to accept help. Past programming can be of service or disservice to us. My past 'spiritual' programming was not 100% serving me at this time, I assure you. Mind chatter would be, 'But I should be able to do this with the help of 'God' and the angels. Why am I not strong enough?' Little did I know on that Monday what was to take place during the coming days.

Wednesday morning dawns and it is a cold, cold day. I do not do cold so I asked Brian if we could have the central heating on for a while, to which he agreed –

well, for five minutes! I went upstairs to get something and, on my return, I was greeted with a banging of walls and doors and shouting at Sylvia about how HE was in charge here and would control things, NOT ME! I avoided contact as best I could and turned the heating off. I was very close to being physically abused as his naughty neurones took over; yes, I admit I was scared. Out to coffee was a good diversion and the rest of the day was a typical in and out of 'neurones' with Sylvia doing her best to be calm and talk calmly at all times to prevent "How dare you speak to me like that? You are always talking like that these days." I try to make him understand that 99.5% of the time I am good, but when very tired words can slip out in a way I do not intend. Eventually, we end up with a hug and reiterating our love to each other. That is indeed a blessing in among all the turmoil of each day.

So we get through Wednesday and deal with the evening/nocturnal sundowning, and Thursday dawns. Day care day. It starts during getting dressed time, where he thinks he can do more than he can, and seems reluctant to go to day care. With loving words and attitude I get compliance until breakfast has successfully been completed and we are talking about something quite mundane. Brian made a comment and I responded. Ooops! Words came out wrong. The tirade of verbal abuse began and he came towards me with an acute 'neurones' look about him. On my guard, I stayed calm as he hit me on the shoulder and continued to shout. I did manage to calm him and he apologised. Some degree of calm then ensued and I took him to the care home. I know I was getting a strong message about letting go and planning full time care. My heart sank with sorrow as I put out a prayer to God and the Angel: 'Dear God, if this is the time to consider a strategy for full time care then the care manager will greet me in reception.' Oh my! There he was when we arrived. I let Brian go through into the unit with someone and the manager quietly asked, "Are you all right Sylvia?"

Through my tears I told him of the episode of the morning and previous day.

"I heard about Monday," he said. "Why don't you go home and get a few clothes together for Brian and let him stay? You cannot go on like this, because one day he could really hurt you – he is a strong man." I cannot fully express the sick feeling I had in the pit of my stomach at that moment. All my plans for care at home were shattered. 'I thought we would have more quality time together as a happily married couple,' went flooding through my mind. 'What am I going to tell him?'

I decided the best thing would be to tell him he needed to stay for a sleep assessment. In spite of my overwhelming grief I knew this was the right thing, and that the circumstances that had occurred were a positive, to show me that I could not continue 'coping' with him at home on my own.

As I drove home feeling absolutely numb and reality being like a dream, tears streamed down my face as the pain of having to 'let go' and leave my darling husband there sank in. On my return home, I recalled the dear friend who had married us, making me promise to call her in times of stress. This was a time where I had to do just that. She came round in a very short while and held me as I sobbed out my grief and pain at what 'naughty neurones' can do. Words of comfort and encouragement that it was the right decision along with a prayer brought calm to my spirit. I felt some inner peace again. Truly I was blessed to have dear friends around me, along with a 'big sister' in Scotland whom I called and who gave me reassurance. After invoking angels and peace later that afternoon, I went to see Brian and break the news. He accepted it fairly well, and I said I would visit him each day. As I left I felt a culmination of relief along with grief to see him sitting there with the other residents: relief that I did not have to carry the burden any longer and grief at what he must be feeling as his wife leaves him. There was a service at our local spiritual church that evening, so I went along to be with friends and break the news, as they had great affection for dear Brian.

Thus began another phase of the Alzheimer's journey.

CHAPTER 17

24/7 Care – A Journey of Its Own!

My first night at home without my darling Brian was indescribably painful, yet mixed with relief, which made me feel guilty that I could not cope. Somehow I was in a dream world. Is this really happening? Did I really go through all that? Yet in among all the emotions that were surfacing, I never felt the need to cry out to God, 'Why me?' At least I could remember our beautiful times together and know I had done my best, I would tell myself whilst pangs of guilt rose up and words from the caveat time echoed in my head: 'You are marrying Brian to live free in his house and dump him in a Care Home.'

Initially I raced in every day to see him, grabbed his washing and took it home to wash and iron it for him within a few days. Every day I was asked how long he would have to stay, and it was not easy having to say I did not know because he was not sleeping at night – actually true as many nights were still spent in the lounge with the night staff. Moods fluctuated with me from day to day and I made very good use of my coaching skills on myself. I decided to re-start the morning yoga and meditation times and begin a routine. One thing was for sure, he was in an excellent care home that stuck rigidly to the day-to-day routine I typed out for them.

My inner spirit and love of my friends and neighbours was strong. Truly I was blessed during this time of major change in our lives. Each day I went in to find him smartly dressed with his hair beautifully done and with a handsome, clean-shaven face, to greet me with hugs and kisses. I worked hard at keeping my emotions in control and invoked the angels to go with me.

Around ten days after his admission, one of the male carers took me to one side and said, "Sylvia, why are you taking Brian's washing home? We can do it here. You are very tired. That is what we are here for. Go to reception and they will tell you how to order some name tags for him." Tears welled up as he reassured me it was all right and how he loved his job and had seen a lot of pain during his time there. I took his advice and stepped into the fear of Brian knowing he had his name on his clothes. The snappy tags were so small he would never notice. It was as if this one suggestion fully reinforced that I was not living out a dream – this was really happening!

Moods with Brian fluctuated during my visits and naturally he would ask me, "What have you done with my home? You've dumped me here!" It took a while to be able to visit him without feeling butterflies in my stomach – even after invoking the protection of the Archangel Michael! If I found a very tetchy mood on arrival it usually changed before I left. Gradually, he began to settle and spoke less and less about the house, which was a relief. However, I have been on a learning curve about what to discuss when visiting: keep conversations light and minimal as the confused neurones can still pick up on current events. On one occasion he asked what I had been doing. Without a thought I told him I had been preparing for that evening's radio show. WRONG! "Oh have you? I always used to come with you. Why can't I come tonight?" I muttered some kind of response and tried to divert the conversation, which thankfully I managed. You see, because of the manifestation of Brian's Alzheimer's it would not be good practice for me to take him out on a visit alone. Behaviour could not be predicted. He could easily get angry and confused about where he should be.

Another time he was not in a good space so I told him I was going to pop and do some shopping and return. "I can come with you," was the response. Thankfully I could safely say it was almost lunchtime, so he needed to stay. I was just realising that when your loved one moves into full time care, it is another journey in itself and brings new challenges:

- Guilt about 'dumping them'
- Guilt around feeling a sense of relief

- Guilt around making changes at home that were necessary
- Guilt about a visiting routine.

This was an interesting behaviour trait for Sylvia, who thought she had dealt with her childhood programmed guilt through religion! A shock too that it was still emerging. Staff at the care home were very supportive and reassured me that Brian was settling in well. Surprise, surprise! He was even going in the bingo sessions – he hated bingo all his life and always said it was a waste of money! Then I hear that he is being persuaded to indulge in exercise! What? Is this my Brian? As Christmas looms he is definitely settling in after around seven weeks stay, and interacting well with everyone. The staff seem to love talking with him and the home manager spends time having a cup of tea with him. They certainly seem to know how to help them adjust. Because Brian is still able to rationalise some things I seem to fall into traps on visits. I talk as if he is the old Brian before the Alzheimer's kicked in. It took me a good three to four months to get it into my head that the 'knowing Sylvia,' and still able to tell her how much he loves her, does not mean that he does not have mostly confused moments.

Other signs of his deterioration were marked communication difficulties. It was like playing the TV game 'What's My Line?' many a time as he struggled to tell me or ask me something, and if I do not understand I am f*****g stupid!" On a bad day I have greeted him and said how much I still love him, to have a curt reply of, "Lies! I don't like lies!" In time this disperses, he is in good spirits and we have a laugh over past times, and then he may say, "How long have I loved you? Can I marry you?" He loves my response to this: "You've loved me for over 17½ years now and you cannot marry me because we are married already!" We then have a good chuckle together and a hug. What a lovely memory I have of this to treasure forever.

Christmas discussions are very sensitively dealt with and I tell him that we can have Christmas where he is, as they will be putting on fun things and it will save us preparing and me cooking. The head chef offers to prepare special food for me, including special Christmas pudding and cake. I begin to feel thoroughly spoilt. Typically, the care home has a Christmas party day and carols, which I attend with Brian, and soon the big day dawns. It was strange being at home alone, but I was beginning to adjust and had made many necessary changes at home by now. I arrived at the home for 11.00 a.m. There was a cup of coffee, biscuits and a singalong before lunch.

Prior to lunch I took Brian into reception and made calls to my family so that he could speak to them. Oh my! Was he then confused about where he should be, or what? I took him into lunch, which was beautifully set out with Christmas tablecloths, crackers and festive menus. We had hardly begun our lunch when the naughty neurones kicked in and I got a real verbal showdown from my man about why weren't we at the house, along with table banging. Then he got up and stormed out of the dining room and had to be calmed down by the nurses. Gradually, during the afternoon, he calmed down and I left him in the early evening in better spirits. On my Boxing Day visit, the nurse in charge called me to the office, saying that I looked tired and did not need to come in every day to see Brian as he was absolutely fine. I agreed to stay away for five days, which generated another very interesting emotional response. When I returned home I felt an emptiness that I described to one of my friends as a feeling of my soul being ripped out. I was going through a major 'letting go' experience. A good old tears release and once again soul-searching and support helped me through. Through my tears yet again, I was able to acknowledge the joy of what we had together in our love and the joyous memories. Inner peace was returning much more quickly these days.

The other impartial lesson one learns or has to acknowledge is that we need at some level to 'let the patient go,' as we cannot take on board what is their life journey. It is guilt that makes us cling to them and try to compensate somehow for what is happening to them. As we grieve someone 'dying' in front of us, we naturally can do the 'what ifs' and 'why,' yet when we acknowledge that this awful journey is part of earthly experience that has to be dealt with as best we can, and by tapping into inner 'reserves' (or as I call it, our higher self), we ease the pain more and more speedily as time goes by.

A visit in the New Year of 2015 by my older sister was great. We had some quality 'girl time' and Brian recognised her on our visits. By now I had adjusted visiting days and am dealing with his lack of time-space recognition well. Sister fell in line with this and enjoyed having Sunday lunch with him, which has become a weekly ritual. The blessing in this? The same quality time with the man I love and no cooking! Brian's blessing is that he gets to have two puddings due to my food intolerance! It is now over five months since full time care had to take place and Brian talks about his room as 'his place.' I have created a structure to visiting and also accompanying him on outings in the minibus. I have adjusted to living at home without him, and am now back on track with my holistic life purpose activities. Yes, there is still more to this journey, but I have learned through it the power of:

- living in the moment
- finding blessings in adversity
- acknowledging personal growth through suffering
- realising that unconditional love allows them to live out their journey of life as it needs to for them
- the joy of forgiveness

- to live out to the very best of our ability what we teach
- know that to 'love thy neighbour' we have to love 'as thyself.'

I am now a much more balanced person and acknowledging the need to take care of me without shame or guilt more fully than I was before.

I would not change a thing that has happened as I reflect on our journey thus far.

To witness my husband grow and both acknowledge and stand in his power with determination to keep the woman he loves has been truly magnificent – to be able to yet again accept that pain is our greatest teacher and can be our greatest awareness of how powerful we are if we deal with pain from our higher self is inspiring. The greatest masters and teachers on our planet have suffered deeply to grow towards expressing their true purpose here on earth.

I truly believe that there is a purpose in our story to help humanity.

Sylvia has embraced her grief and allowed it to further teach and empower her.

May you be able to find even a glimmer of inner peace and joy as you journey through your life.

What follows next is how we did our very best to integrate holistic methods into this journey.

CHAPTER 18

Integration – A Holistic Approach

From a pure nursing background, I have integrated to working in the holistic area as a transformational coach and healer. Once I knew what diagnosis we were dealing with in respect of my husband, I began to research on the internet. The consultant knew I was a Reiki master teacher/healer and because Brian was so young – only 62 years of age when formally diagnosed – he was open to me trying whatever I felt might help hold back his progress. This is when Sylvia is great for her internet skills and computer skill knowledge, as well as her basic knowledge covering the importance of supplements in one's diet in this modern age, where our foods are so tampered with and genetically modified. My mission now was to find specific food-based natural substances to help his brain function plateau for as long as possible.

It has been widely known in natural medicine circles the benefits of Omega oils to help brain tissues, as the brain is made up primarily of fatty tissues. This was on our list of extras, alongside his drug treatment of Aricept 10 mgs per day. I am not going to specify a dosage here; let's leave you to do your own research, and see the references at the end of the book.

For at least a decade or two now, the power of antioxidants has also been proven to prevent oxidation in tissues and promote overall health and disease prevention. These had been a part of my daily food supplementation and Brian was now keen to add in whatever I felt would help. His trust in me touched me greatly, not only that but he expressed deep gratitude for what I was doing. I felt that it was the least I could do for the man I had married and so deeply loved. Vitamin C is a simple antioxidant plus there are also combinations, concentrated natural drinks and capsules available.

With any supplementation, pure organic is recommended, as it will be totally free of pesticides and include only certain natural preservatives in accordance with legislation having incorporated Omega oils and antioxidants into Brian's healthy living routine. I was now encouraging a diet of fresh natural, simple foods and drinks and as advised by the consultant on an alcohol free drinks regime. Let me emphasise here that in no way did I force my alternative approaches on my dear man, but he now believed in the power of natural ways to improve health and became open minded.

Alongside dietary improvements he was also being offered energy healing to help re-balance his energies and hopefully generate some improvement. Somewhere inside of me with my beliefs I was hoping that one day a miraculous recovery would take place. However, the story told shows that at the very least we were able to contain things for a while. If the diagnosis would have been made sooner, who knows how much we could have held the disease back? Still, I also believe in our purpose here on earth and that Brian's purpose must also be allowed to play out within his choices.

As I 'Googled' and 'YouTubed' I found many so-called 'cures' for Alzheimer's, but wanted to research natural help. Then one day I stumbled on a video that had been put up by the son of a gentleman with quite severe Alzheimer's. He had heard of the benefits of coconut oil and decided to try it on his father. Amazingly there were quite dramatic improvements in various ways. One example was how he had needed feeding and was unable to lift a drink up himself, but after a week or two of being given organic raw coconut oil he picked up a cup and started drinking. Other improvements were also reported. I managed to track him down and spoke with him at length. This was in 2012 and he was then working to raise funds for an in-depth trial here in the UK. He suggested I track down a Dr. Mary Newport in the USA and read her book on the benefits of coconut oil with dementia and Alzheimer's. This I did and found her information extremely interesting. She was a neonatal consultant for premature babies and they used intravenous medium chain triglycerides to stimulate neurone production in the babies' brain tissue as it developed. Her husband also had Alzheimer's disease, so there was a personal reason for her research. She figures that if M.C.Ts. helped premature babies' brains surely they must be able to help Alzheimer's disease sufferers. As someone with a nursing background, I could resonate with her and studied her findings and results with her husband. She was even seen on American TV talking about coconut oil. I managed to personally track her down and email and phone communication took place for a short time, which I valued from a busy woman. As you can imagine, with Brian's agreement I introduced coconut oil and M.C.T. oil into his dietary regime by adding it to his porridge every morning, plus a little over the vegetables in the evening. Cooking was now with coconut oil, as it is said by some authorities to be the only oil that is non toxic on heating.

There were some improvements with Brian's cognitive skills for a short time and he did seem to plateau for a good while. However, the damage to his brain shown in the P.E.T. scans would challenge even the very best coconut oil, I hate to say. These were the main add-ins to a healthy diet for him, and he still has his coconut and M.C. T. oils in the care home as they are under the umbrella of foodstuffs. Other supplements are not allowed as they are not able to be prescribed. It takes patience and creativity to get his Aricept into him.

I also believe that perhaps unresolved emotional issues could affect brain functions as old pains and experiences are buried and not dealt with in a positive way. Who knows? Now that science is able to capture thoughts on a computer, we have an almost bottomless pit of possibilities that are worth considering.

I have recently stumbled on – or not – books by a Dr Richard S. Issacson of the USA, who is a Professor of Clinical Neurology with a specific interest in Alzheimer's disease. He writes about some very interesting evidence-based material as well as having penned a book with dietary recommendations for the prevention and treatment of Alzheimer's. As drug companies search for a cure, let us also keep searching for mother nature's answers.

My philosophy?

- Feed your brain
- Live a healthy lifestyle
- Be in the moment at all times.

CHAPTER 19

Some Suggestions from Sylvia

Based on our journey and my experience as a carer, I thought I would give some simple suggestions from my own experience that may help others. In no particular order, just as they flow:

- Try and get a diagnosis as early as possible
- As soon as you have suspicions, start a healthy eating and supplement programme
- Do your own early research: good old Google and YouTube
- Listen to your own intuition and only follow the good advice of others if it sits right with you and your circumstances
- Remember that your journey is unique. Do not let others try to govern. With the general concept lies the individual manifestation and quirks of the disease based on past life experiences and the patient's perception of self, and how they relate to the world
- Always try to see things from their painful,

frustrating world, especially in the early days of diagnosis
- Anger is more often than not frustration until confusional symptoms increase
- A daily routine helps with memory retention, and task setting is a big help
- Do not change things around. They will have a programmed memory of where things are in the home and where furniture is. This is important if they are manifesting posterior cortex atrophy
- Use contrasting colours for ease of recognition. I bought a cheap set of crockery in Argos plus coloured handled cutlery and bright coloured place mats. White cups and saucers merge, and plain white mug handles are challenging to find
- Let them do as much as possible for as long as possible, even if they 'fumble' and 'swear.' Just be mindful of the occasional item flying past, like a box, a shoe, or even socks and underwear!
- As they progress, subtly cut up foods and try to serve dishes that are easy to manage. If in a restaurant, do not be shy to ask for food to be cut up a little – saves a good deal of angry neurones in public
- Be prepared to live more untidily on this journey and expect things like toothpaste to be everywhere in the bathroom
- If possible, have a wipe clean surface in the toilet and bathroom to make it easy to deal with male

mishaps with 'pointing Percy at the porcelain!'
- Let them struggle before you 'muscle in' to help, because they think they can still do things
- Use humour wherever possible: it helps dissipate frustration
- Bear in mind that helpful professional advice will rarely be taken by them: "I don't need help"
- Remember that you too are on this journey, so find ways to nurture yourself if possible
- Prevent crisis situations wherever possible and accept help
- They may sometimes be more compliant with people they know than strangers at home
- Re-adjust routines according to their manifestations and challenges subtly so they become compliant for you
- Do not expect long attention spans
- Music is a great diversional trigger
- Have courage when out to openly get help for them without it being overly obvious
- Acknowledge that you will not get it right all the time and do not beat yourself up about it
- Remember the mantra and breathing – "I choose peace" – practice this regularly
- Do not try to convince them that things are in their best interests as they will still believe 'they know best'
- Like a child, allow them to have to accept things

through their own struggles to cope
- Place pictures around you that remind you of the good times
- Create your own memory album – even of times in the care home. This helps with adjustment at different stages
- Find at least one blessing in amongst the challenging days – it will keep you sane
- Call helplines if you feel desperate. A few minutes offload and/or tears will be a release and give you the strength to carry on
- If they are 'sundowners' then try to take a power nap when they drift off. When nursing I could crash out for ten minutes and be refreshed
- Use focused relaxation to rest the body – sit comfortably, relax your breathing and imagine yourself in a pink bubble, and silently say, 'I am at peace – all is well'
- Say the above Mantra every time you need a loo visit where, for a minute or two, you are alone. In fact, use it as frequently as you need
- Minimise caffeine and sugar in the diet to help keep them as calm as possible. If you like baking, substitute hard fats for coconut oil. Recipes are plentiful now on the internet.

In Summary

Although a tortuous and challenging journey thus far, I can honestly say that I have grown as a person to an even greater level of reaching the power of living from the 'real person' who resides within us and will guide us in our actions and decisions if we listen.

For Sylvia the mind follows on to logically create the right action and positive thoughts from the inspired self. Guilt lessens as we realise that no-one is in a position to judge another's life journey. No-one has the right to say, "This is the way" or "That is the way" without us finding out for ourself if that course of action or interpretation of information sits well with our beliefs and values.

I have come to realise that if there is some degree of compliance from the person you are caring for, and whatever action is taken is in their best interest, and yours, then guilt does not have to be an option.

I have also learned to count the blessings along the way and to treasure the joyous times and precious moments we do share.

References

Dr Mary Newport MD – *Alzheimer's Disease – What if There Was a Cure?* Available from Amazon.
Her Research and her Husband's response with Coconut Oil. Check out YouTube for up to date information from her.
Dr Richard S Issacson MD – *Alzheimer's Treatment – Alzheimer's Prevention* and *the Alzheimer's Diet.*
Alzheimer's Society – www.alzheimers.org.uk and find your country
Dementia Aware Facebook Page – https:www.facebook.com/groups/250325295027020/
Carers Support – search online for your area
Natural approaches to Alzheimer's – an internet search will bring up information for you to sift through
Samaritans – http://www.samaritans.org/
Amazon for Books and Kindle Reading on Alzheimer's and Dementia